OXFORD MODERN LANGUAGES AND LITERATURE MONOGRAPHS

The Doctor–Patient Relationship and the Nineteenth-Century French Novel

SARAH JONES

OXFORD
UNIVERSITY PRESS

OXFORD
UNIVERSITY PRESS

Great Clarendon Street, Oxford, OX2 6DP,
United Kingdom

Oxford University Press is a department of the University of Oxford.
It furthers the University's objective of excellence in research, scholarship,
and education by publishing worldwide. Oxford is a registered trade mark of
Oxford University Press in the UK and in certain other countries

Published in the United States of America by Oxford University Press
198 Madison Avenue, New York, NY 10016, United States of America

British Library Cataloguing in Publication Data

Data available

Library of Congress Control Number: 2023941591

ISBN 9780198893790

DOI: 10.1093/oso/9780198893790.001.0001

Printed and bound in the UK by
Clays Ltd, Elcograf S.p.A.

Acknowledgements

This book began life as my doctoral thesis, submitted at the University of Oxford in 2019, and as such my greatest thanks go to those who supported this project during its early stages. I am grateful to the Clore Duffield Foundation which funded my doctoral study at Oxford, as well as to the Gapper Charitable Trust which awarded me the Sévigné studentship for my Masters study at King's College London. I would like to thank Oriel College, for the academic and financial support given to me during my time as a student there, and my examiners who meticulously and generously read my thesis at various stages: Andrew Counter, Hannah Thompson, Caroline Warman, and Jennifer Yee. I am also thankful to the community of scholars in nineteenth-century French studies and beyond who welcomed me into their fold. Finally, I am grateful to all my colleagues and peers at Oxford and its constituent colleges who read, supported, and encouraged my work, and helped me find a sense of perspective and joy.

Parts of Chapter One appeared as 'Zola's Fortunate Man: Rereading Doctor Pascal as a Country Doctor' in 'Critical French Medical Humanities' in *Essays in French Literature and Culture*, 58 (2021). Very early forms of Chapter Two appeared as '"Jeune fille qui ne pleure pas son oiseau mort": Female Puberty in Stendhal's *Lamiel*' in *Nineteenth-Century French Studies*, 50 (2021–22) and as 'Stendhal's Consumptive Heroine: *Lamiel* and Tuberculosis' in *French Studies*, 77 (2023). An earlier version of Chapter Three appeared as 'Écrire le corps cholérique dans *Lélia* de George Sand' in *Romantisme*, 198 (2022). I am grateful to the editors and readers of these journals and edited volumes with their help with these articles. My thanks also go to the anonymous readers at Oxford University Press whose kind suggestions helped shape my thesis into a monograph.

Contents

Note on Translations

All translations from French into English are my own unless otherwise stated.

Introduction
Literary Medical Relationships and Encounters

Reading Medicine

Paris, 1819. Two students, one studying law and the other medicine, argue about how to care for their neighbour who has fallen critically ill. The medical student suggests that they should apply a mustard plaster, acting as a counterirritant to inflame the skin and distract the patient from his physical and emotional suffering. Deeply unsettled by his friend's enthusiasm for medical interventions, as well as 'fait[s] scientifique[s]' ['scientific facts'] more generally, the law student complains that 'je serai donc le seul à soigner ce pauvre vieillard par affection' ['I'll be the only one who heals this poor old man with affection'].[1] The medical student is offended and, to differentiate himself from his more clinically minded peers, he points out that 'Les médecins qui ont exercé ne voient que la maladie, moi, je vois encore le malade' ['Doctors who have practised only see the illness, but I still see the patient'].[2] The scene reminds the reader that medicine is always being negotiated: there is no singular way that doctors should treat their patients and, as such, caregivers and those they care for continually debate what medicine should be.

This scene from *Le Père Goriot* evokes a significant change in the structure and focus of medicine in the nineteenth century. Historians of medicine generally see eighteenth-century medicine as organized around the patient and argue that nineteenth-century medicine assumed a greater interest in the nature of disease on the level of cells and tissues.[3] As such, Bianchon's use of the verb *voir* inevitably brings to mind the nineteenth-century *regard medical* ['medical gaze'], the penetrating, examining vision that doctors apply to the patient, their body, and their illness. Foucault defines medical vision both literally (the doctor sees his patient, who is both subject and object of study) and conceptually. The development of

[1] Honoré de Balzac, *Le Père Goriot*, ed. by Félicien Marceau (Paris: Gallimard, 1971), p. 339. All translations given in square brackets are my own.

[2] Ibid.

[3] For a summary of the historiographical changes that led to this characterization, see Laurence Brockliss and Colin Jones, *The Medical World of Early Modern France* (Oxford: Clarendon Press, 1997), pp. 1–6.

The Doctor–Patient Relationship and the Nineteenth-Century French Novel. Sarah Jones, Oxford University Press.
 DOI: 10.1093/oso/9780198893790.003.0001

the medical clinic, and its particular form of medical vision, he argues, redefined and reorganized medicine as an empirical field of knowledge.[4]

But in *Le Père Goriot*, 'voir' is also used figuratively: Bianchon does not only mean that he literally sees the patient, but that he recognizes and acknowledges Goriot's embodied experience and the depth of his physical and emotional pain. Rather than only debating how to treat Goriot medically, the two students discuss how to treat him interpersonally. Bianchon attempts to create a different medical relationship to the one that we may anticipate, and that seems to be cultivated by his own medical education. Rather than diagnosing and curing Goriot, Bianchon wants to heal him through recognition and understanding, 'par affection' as Rastignac states. Although Bianchon is not yet a fully qualified doctor, the passage poses important questions about the importance of the interpersonal dynamic between doctor and patient, its bearing on the practice of medicine, and its role within the literary representation of medicine during the nineteenth century. It is these questions that the present monograph seeks to answer.

In this volume I argue that medicine is depicted as more than a science in nineteenth-century novels: it is seen as a form of practice, an ongoing negotiation between doctor and patient, between expert and sufferer, between observer and observed. Focusing on literary portrayals of the doctor–patient relationship, which I define as the ongoing interpersonal connection between doctor and patient, draws out the fluidity and dynamism of nineteenth-century medical practice. The literary medical relationship is not just a facet of or vehicle for medicine, but instead is a form of practice and knowledge that is conceptualized, imagined, indeed created, by the nineteenth-century novel. The doctor–patient relationship draws attention to the interpersonal, embodied, and experiential dimension of medicine and illness that hovers on the borders between life and death. As the previous passage from *Le Père Goriot* highlights, questions of power dynamics, the status and function of language, and the role of aesthetics influence the form, function, and meaning of the doctor–patient relationship in the novels in which it appears. The present study interrogates the doctor–patient relationship by configuring it as an object of knowledge itself and thereby as a potential subject of study and criticism.

The term 'doctor–patient relationship' finds its roots in the medical humanities, a field that was originally conceived in the 1950s with the intention of humanizing the medical sciences. In the early decades of its inception, the medical humanities focused on dichotomies which provided fundamental structures within medicine, such as that between doctor and patient. As such, the doctor–patient relationship was central to the medical humanities, serving as both the field's founding concept and primary object of study. The structure of the doctor–patient relationship

[4] Michel Foucault, *Naissance de la clinique* (Paris: Presses universitaires de France, 2017).

may seem to enforce a false binary between doctor and patient, or to create an imagined hierarchy that sees the latter subjugated to the former's authority but, in this study, I aim to demonstrate that the doctor–patient relationship, and literary portrayals of it, are always in a state of flux. This argument echoes that of Anne Whitehead and Angela Woods whose landmark study heralded the beginning of the critical medical humanities, in which the medical humanities aligns itself with critical turns in other disciplines in order to address 'more theoretically charged questions'.[5] They argue that the critical medical humanities' focus on 'mobility, fluidity, and movement' in the practice of medicine allows for a multitude of 'creative boundary-crossing' that transcends the conventional categories of doctor and patient, science and art, illness and narrative.[6] Approaches to representations of medicine in nineteenth-century French literature are becoming increasingly influenced by the critical medical humanities and the present study revisits the doctor–patient relationship with these arguments and approaches in mind.[7] Rather than abandoning this founding concept of the medical humanities, I seek to turn a critical eye to the doctor–patient relationship by examining its form and function within the nineteenth-century French novel. The present study thus sees medicine as a form of dynamic interpersonal practice that is open to both idealization and satire; whose binary and hierarchical elements can be entrenched or subverted; and whose relationship to narrative, metaphor, and plot may be questioned.

To add further dimension to the concept of the medical relationship, I propose the doctor–patient encounter as a second, competing paradigm within literature. The nineteenth-century novel treats medical encounters differently from relationships. Whereas relationships are idealized, enduring interpersonal connections, encounters are represented as dynamic and unpredictable moments within these relationships that can disrupt, subvert, or even invert, the premises on which the relationship is predicated. Let us briefly move away from literature to take a real-life example of this process. A patient may respect the family doctor who has treated them for their entire life. Yet a disappointing medical encounter, such as one where the doctor fails to acknowledge a patient's pain, may cause the patient to question the doctor's authority, subtly altering the balance of power within their

[5] Anne Whitehead and Angela Woods, 'Introduction', in *The Edinburgh Companion to the Critical Medical Humanities*, ed. by Anne Whitehead and Angela Woods (Edinburgh: Edinburgh University Press, 2016), pp. 1–32 (p. 8).

[6] Ibid., p. 8.

[7] Recent interventions in this burgeoning sub-field of French studies include Steven Wilson, 'Introduction: Connecting Medicine and Religion in Modern French Literature', ed. by Steven Wilson, *Modern and Contemporary France*, L'Imaginaire médico-religieux: Modern French Literary Perspectives, 28.4 (2020), 357–64; Enda McCaffrey and Steven Wilson, 'Introduction: Death and/as Relationality', in *French Thanatology*, ed. by Enda McCaffrey and Steven Wilson (special issue, *L'Esprit Créateur*, 61.1 (2021)), 1–12; Enda McCaffrey and Áine Larkin, Introduction to *The Critical Medical Humanities*, ed. by Enda McCaffrey and Áine Larkin (special issue, *Essays in French Literature and Culture*, 58 (2021)), 3–14.

enduring interpersonal relationship. The medical encounter is therefore a potentially disruptive space, subverting the power dynamic on which it is founded. However, as we shall see in Chapter Four, the disruptive potential of medical encounters can itself be harnessed to build a new form of the doctor–patient relationship.

These conceptions of the medical relationship and encounter are not, however, antithetical to one another or indeed mutually exclusive. Instead, they are inherently interconnected in the nineteenth-century French novel insofar as interpersonal relationships are composed of a series of encounters, and encounters are often the products of longstanding relationships. As such, there is significant slippage between the medical relationship and the encounter. Moreover, the degree of slippage between these two terms is neither stable nor predictable. As we will see in Chapter Three, Balzac's *La Peau de chagrin* shows us a medical encounter that seems to encapsulate and speak to the broader medical relationship within which the encounter is located. In contrast, the medical encounters of *L'Interdiction* are almost entirely abstracted from the doctor–patient relationship. Medical encounters, and their connection to the medical relationships of which they are components, are thus multivalent in the French novel. But what reading these encounters into our depiction of literary representations of medicine allows us is an understanding of how practical medicine is understood by authors to occupy different forms of space and time and that the function of medicine may change depending on these. These conditions determine the opportunity for subjugation or disruption on the part of the medical encounter.

By analysing the concept of the doctor–patient relationship within the nineteenth-century French novel, I assert a vision of medicine as a form of practice, experience, and interpersonal negotiation. I compare literary texts to eighteenth- and nineteenth-century medical texts in order to throw new light on how literary and medical writers understood and represented medicine. My historicist approach reflects the different historical meanings and functions of medicine and science after the 1789 Revolution. For example, in the 1798 edition of the *Dictionnaire de l'Académie française*, *science* is defined according to three levels: firstly, 'Connoissance qu'on a de quelque chose' ['Knowledge one has of something']; secondly, 'Connoissance certaine et évidente des choses' ['Certain and evident knowledge of things']; and, finally, 'La connoissance de toutes les choses dans lesquelles on est bien instruit' ['Knowledge of all the things about which one has been taught'].[8] It is not until 1932 that *science* was defined by the rational and experimental processes that we now associate with science, although a generalist version of the word still took precedence: 'Connaissance exacte qu'on a de quelque chose. [...] Système de connaissances rationnelles ou

[8] *Le Dictionnaire de l'Académie française*, vol. 2 (Paris: J. J. Smits et Ce, 1798), s.v. 'science'.

expérimentales sur un objet déterminé'.[9] Before the twentieth century, then, *science* is best understood as a broad and diverse form of knowledge (or indeed knowledges). My intention here is not to minimize the medical advances made during the nineteenth century, which are numerous and self-evident, but instead to question the teleological narrative that posits medicine as becoming straightforwardly scientific thanks to these developments.[10]

When examining the representation of medical science in the nineteenth-century novel, it is therefore crucial to abandon twenty-first-century expectations of a form of science that has become wholly scientific in its outlook, approaches, and forms of knowledge. Gaston Bachelard, for example, illustrates how science is constantly negotiated and refined: '[e]n fait, on connaît *contre* une connaissance antérieure, en détruisant des connaissances mal faites' ['in fact, one knows *against* a previous form of knowledge, by destroying knowledge that was badly put together'].[11] Overcoming these obstacles undermines science's claims to the *réel* since '[l]e réel n'est jamais "ce qu'on pourrait croire" mais il est toujours ce qu'on aurait dû penser' ['the real is never "what may be believed" but is always what should have been thought of'].[12]. By reading literary texts alongside a range of illnesses, including both infectious and non-communicable disease, I point towards the determining structures of medical knowledge, authority, and practice. My research thus builds on work by scholars in nineteenth-century French studies, such as Larry Duffy who explores the incorporation of medical knowledge and discourses into Flaubert's and Zola's works.[13] Furthermore, the breadth and diversity of the dictionary definition of *science* suggest the importance of challenging the supposed critical dichotomy between science and art, the two fields between which medicine is classically understood to be torn. Reading across the conventional boundary between science and art allows us to perceive, as Sophie Leroy outlines, the permeability of the frontiers between these disciplines.[14]

Beyond the doctor–patient relationship and encounter, four other concepts recur in this volume: the theme and role of (medical) vision, the functioning of medical metaphors, the construction and destruction of medical plots, and

[9] *Le Dictionnaire de l'Académie française*, vol. 2 (Paris: Hachette, 1935), s.v. 'science'.

[10] Numerous advances were made in a number of medical fields including pharmaceuticals (the development of aspirin during the 1830s and the use of quinine to treat malaria in 1820), surgery (the use of nitric oxide as an anaesthetic in 1844 and the first open-heart surgery in 1895), hygiene (most notably the use of antiseptic from 1867 and the development of germ theory from the 1850s), medical technology (such as the invention of the stethoscope in 1816) and the development of vaccination programmes against smallpox from 1813 onwards.

[11] Gaston Bachelard, *La Formation de l'esprit scientifique: contribution à une psychanalyse de la connaissance objective* (Paris: Librairie J. Vrin, 2000), pp. 15–16.

[12] Ibid., p. 15.

[13] Larry Duffy, *Flaubert, Zola, and the Incorporation of Disciplinary Knowledge* (Basingstoke, New York: Palgrave Macmillan, 2015).

[14] Sophie Leroy, 'Introduction', in *Medicine and Maladies: Representing Affliction in Nineteenth-Century France*, ed. by Sophie Leroy (Leiden: Brill, 2018), pp. 1–15 (p. 1).

the importance of identity and power within the medical relationship. As Bianchon's use of the word 'voir' in *Le Père Goriot* suggests, the nature of vision is central to understanding nineteenth-century depictions of medicine, in particular its relationship to patients, illness, and the development of nineteenth-century literature. However, I argue that this medical vision is not merely a structuring concept that understands the patient and contributes to the structuring of medicine, but that medical vision includes more abstract elements that, for example, dovetail with idealism and paternalism. Moving beyond the analogy between medical and realist vision, I illustrate how figurative language, particularly medical and corporeal metaphors, is relied upon in medical scenes and during the doctor–patient relationship. This study throws new light on both the position of medicine within nineteenth-century literary plots, and the plots that structure the representation of medicine in those novels. The literary depiction of the body is a recurring theme, and I particularly focus on how female patients are represented in terms of corporeality and embodied experience. Questions regarding gender, particularly femininity, coalesce around the doctor–patient relationship, rendering the medical relationship and encounter important sites for understanding the politics of identity and its representation in nineteenth-century literature. In short, from this study, the doctor–patient relationship and encounter emerge as two important paradigms in which nineteenth-century French novelists sought to understand the practice of medicine within the broader context of medical discourse.

The Medical Humanities and the Doctor–Patient Relationship

Conceived in the United States of America in the 1950s to offer a diverse humanist dimension to medical school training, the medical humanities draw on the humanities, arts, and social sciences, putting them in dialogue with conventional medical pedagogy. The doctor–patient relationship was one of the central foci of the first significant wave of the medical humanities, and it was understood to be central to the practice and experience of medicine. Michael Balint's 1957 work, *The Doctor, His Patient, and the Illness*, inaugurated the medical humanities and sought to examine 'certain processes within the doctor–patient relationship [...] which caused both the patient and the doctor unnecessary suffering'.[15] The common situation of a doctor attempting to locate a patient's problem only gave rise to the patient's disappointment and anxiety since the prescribed tests would return inconclusive or negative results since, he suggests, the patient's problem lies elsewhere. Balint writes that 'At the outset, I had some idea that, psychologically, much

[15] Michael Balint, *The Doctor, His Patient, and the Illness*, with an 'Introduction' by John A. Balint (Edinburgh: Churchill Livingstone, 2000), p. 4.

more happens in general practice between patient and doctor than is discussed in the traditional textbooks': namely, that the medical relationship was an opportunity for the doctor to locate the psychological origin of the patient's physical ailment.[16]

There have also been significant attempts to provide models for the doctor–patient relationship, which seek to both explain different modes of medical practice as well as to provide aspirational models for practitioners. Thomas Szasz and Marc Hollender outline three models of the physician–patient relationship defined by each participant's respective roles: activity–passivity, guidance–cooperation, and mutual participation.[17] One of the medical humanities' primary occupations was to use the doctor–patient relationship to characterize medicine as a shaped by the patient as well as the doctor. The most important way in which this aim was pursued was through a new emphasis on the patient's personal experience of illness and medicine. Arthur Kleinman, an early pioneer of the field, argues that the Foucauldian isolation of disease from the patient equates to the alienation of the patient from their doctor, thereby also removing the doctor from their own caregiving role which is best understood holistically.[18] Writers such as Kleinman, Oliver Sacks, and Arthur Frank thus all argue that, in order to reinstate these intra- and interpersonal connections, the doctor should begin his medical practice by first caring for the patient's story, a theme to which I return later.[19] Ezekiel Emanuel and Linda Emanuel's 1992 reconfiguration of these models (into the categories paternalistic, informative, interpretive, and deliberative) continues to influence medical education in the UK and elsewhere today.[20] More broadly, in the twenty-first century, scholars maintain an enduring interest in the importance of interpersonal and relational elements such as trust, knowledge, regard, and loyalty to the doctor–patient relationship as well as the patient's health outcomes.[21] The doctor–patient relationship therefore continues to be an important way to conceptualize medical practice and is subject to reappraisals such as that by the general practitioner Peter Bailey who seeks to 'restore the authority' of the medical consultation.[22]

[16] Ibid., pp. 2–3.

[17] Thomas S. Szasz and M. H. Hollender, 'A Contribution to the Philosophy of Medicine: The Basic Models of the Doctor–Patient Relationship', *AMA Archives of Internal Medicine*, 97.5 (1956), 585.

[18] Arthur Kleinman, *The Illness Narratives: Suffering, Healing and the Human Condition* (New York: Basic Books, 1988), pp. 60–80.

[19] Ibid., p. 253. See also Oliver Sacks, *The Man Who Mistook His Wife for a Hat* (London: Picador, 1986), p. 105 and Arthur W. Frank, *The Wounded Storyteller: Body, Illness, and Ethics* (Chicago, IL: University of Chicago Press, 2013), p. xix. My summary here builds on that of Josie Billington, see Josie Billington, *Is Literature Healthy?* (Oxford: Oxford University Press, 2016), pp. 51–3.

[20] Ezekiel J. Emanuel and Linda Emanuel, 'Four Models of the Physician–Patient Relationship', *JAMA: The Journal of the American Medical Association*, 267.16 (1992), 2221.

[21] Fallon E. Chipidza, Rachel S. Wallwork, and Theodore A. Stern, 'Impact of the Doctor–Patient Relationship', *The Primary Care Companion For CNS Disorders*, 17.5 (2015).

[22] Peter Bailey, *The New Doctor, Patient, Illness Model: Restoring the Authority of the GP Consultation* (London: Radcliffe Publishing, 2014).

Despite its grounding in the twentieth century, the medical humanities' concept of the doctor–patient relationship can be productively applied to the nineteenth century. As we have already seen, science was not defined according to strictly scientific terms during this period: similarly, medicine was also not considered as the straightforward application of scientific knowledge. For example, in the 1835 edition of the *Dictionnaire de l'Académie française*, medicine was defined as primarily art which aimed to heal the sick: 'L'art qui enseigne les moyens de conserver la santé, et de traiter les maladies' ['The art which teaches the means of preserving health and of curing illnesses'].[23] In the same edition of the *Dictionnaire*, the second definition of medicine given is 'Celle qui se pratique auprès du lit des malades' ['That which is practised at patients' bedsides'].[24] In this definition, the importance of practice to medicine, as well as its bedside location, confirms that medicine is as much the interpersonal relationship and interaction between doctor and patient as it is the knowledge of human health and illness. These definitions of medicine remind us that although medicine may draw on a body of scientific knowledge, the practice of medicine in the nineteenth century was understood as an ongoing interpersonal negotiation between doctor and patient.

The publication of the *Edinburgh Companion to the Critical Medical Humanities* in 2016 heralded a dramatic shift in approaches to the medical humanities by inaugurating the term 'critical medical humanities'. Whereas first-wave medical humanities was structured around oppositional binaries, such as that between doctor and patient, the critical medical humanities instead highlight the inherently dynamic and fluid nature of medicine that allows for new forms of knowledge to emerge.[25] The critical medical humanities engenders an expansion of the previous focus on the doctor–patient relationship to include contexts and experiences of health, illness, and medicine beyond the 'primal scene of the clinical encounter'.[26] It also calls for scholars to acknowledge the entangled nature of the academic disciplines of arts, humanities, and sciences, which contribute to a 'biomedical culture'.[27] The present volume attempts to respond to these calls. By contextualizing literary depictions of medicine with contemporaneous medical sources, I expand our understanding of the medical and scientific backdrop to the nineteenth-century French novel. Throughout, I emphasize that the boundaries between medicine and arts were not only porous but inherently dynamic: in nineteenth-century literature, medicine was conceived as a practice that transcended or even collapsed the borders between science and art. This study also marks a conceptual return to the doctor–patient relationship. Revisiting this cornerstone of first-wave medical humanities, I treat critically the concept of the medical relationship from

[23] *Le Dictionnaire de l'Académie française*, vol. 2 (Paris: Didot, 1835), s.v. 'médecine'.
[24] Ibid.
[25] Whitehead and Woods, 'Introduction', p. 8.
[26] Ibid., p. 8.
[27] Ibid., p. 2.

the perspective of the critical medical humanities and of French literary studies. The doctor–patient relationship is far from straightforwardly asymmetric, hierarchical, and binary; throughout this study we encounter literary episodes that disrupt, subvert, and even invert these expectations. When the doctor–patient relationship is depicted with the conventional power dynamic of a patient subjugated to the doctor's superior power and knowledge, such as we will see in Chapters One and Four, I examine to what extent a conventionally hierarchical or paternal doctor–patient relationship is in fact a product of idealism and of idealization. I argue that novelistic depictions of medicine widened the definition of the medical relationship beyond that of one doctor and their patient, to include social and political contexts, plural or multiple doctor–patient relationships, as well as characters who perform healing roles and whose functions thus imitate those of professional medical practitioners. This broader definition of the doctor–patient relationship throws light on how early studies in the medical humanities assume that a doctor would be white, male, middle-class, middle-aged, and (for the most part) not living with a disability or chronic illness. Given the exclusion of marginalized groups from professional medical practice during the nineteenth century, these characteristics are also pervasive in the medical novels of the era. However, I demonstrate how the dynamism and fluidity inherent to the doctor–patient relationship and encounter disrupts the stable identity of the doctor, questioning the privileges that he enjoys. The present study thus paves the way for a broader understanding of other forms of medical or healing roles in the nineteenth-century novel such as midwives, nurses, and dentists, as well as other caregivers in the home and wider community.

Introducing the term 'doctor–patient encounter' to my discussion of the medical relationship broadens our understanding of the literary representation of medicine as polylithic. I define the doctor–patient encounter as the highly charged meeting between doctor and patient, often depicted in the nineteenth-century novel as a bedside encounter between physician and patient. The term 'doctor–patient encounter' is used in the medical humanities, but is often conflated with 'doctor–patient relationship'.[28] Indeed, studies with a declared interest in the doctor–patient relationship habitually focus on the medical interview rather than the enduring interpersonal relationship between doctor and patient that continues outside the consultation.[29] The medical encounter necessarily 'flows' from the doctor–patient relationship[30] since relationships begin by an encounter and are perpetuated through them, but in

[28] Michael Dunn, 'At the Moral Margins of the Doctor–Patient Relationship', *Journal of Medical Ethics*, 45.3 (2019), 149–50.

[29] For an example of this usage, see Susan Dorr Goold and Mack Lipkin, 'The Doctor–Patient Relationship: Challenges, Opportunities, and Strategies', *Journal of General Internal Medicine*, 14.S1 (1999), S26–33.

[30] Chipidza, Wallwork, and Stern, 'Impact of the Doctor–Patient Relationship'.

the present study I illustrate how medical relationships and encounters can be productively treated as competing, yet inherently interdependent, concepts. I do this by demonstrating how nineteenth-century authors drew out the encounter as possessing a different ideological character when embedded within a novel.

One of the central themes in this study is that nineteenth-century novels identify the contrast between the idealized doctor–patient relationship, on the one hand, and the doctor–patient encounter on the other. Even today, we may imagine that the doctor–patient relationship is built on trust; but we may find that our actual meeting with the doctor may disappoint our expectations with the result of increased feelings of uncertainty, isolation, and even physical or mental harm. Indeed, the concept of the doctor–patient encounter may speak more convincingly to many patients' experience of medicine: although all NHS patients are appointed a personal GP, this doctor performs an oversight role and patients now have the right, and may prefer, to see another practitioner. This form of care means that some patients may see their relationship with general medicine as a series of discrete encounters with different individuals, rather than an enduring relationship.[31] Whilst insisting on the connection between the doctor–patient relationship and encounter, the contrast between the term structures the chapters of this book: Chapters One and Four focus on the idealization of the doctor–patient relationship; Chapters Two and Three engage with more episodic encounters that illustrate the extent to which the nineteenth-century novel foregrounds the failed expectations of the idealized doctor–patient relationship. In this way, this study responds to Anna Elsner's calls to examine how literature undoes the medical paternalism inherent in the doctor–patient relationship by, firstly, examining how this medical paternalism is the product of idealism and, secondly, illustrating how the conventional power dynamics that it creates can be resisted.[32]

The critical medical humanities maintain an interest in expanding its focus from the modern and contemporary English-speaking world in order to include a greater diversity of global, linguistic, and historical perspectives on the field. In his recent study of nineteenth-century depictions of syphilis, Steven Wilson points out the tendency of early studies in the medical humanities to focus, firstly, on Anglophone contexts and, secondly, on twentieth-century examples and practices.[33] The present study responds to Wilson's observation by foregrounding the dynamism and urgency of questions about the progress and practice of

[31] British Medical Association, 'Requirement for All Patients to Have a Named GP', *BMA*, 7 September 2020, <https://www.bma.org.uk/advice-and-support/gp-practices/managing-your-practice-list/requirement-for-all-patients-to-have-a-named-gp>.

[32] Anna Magdalena Elsner, 'Beyond Medical Paternalism: Undoing the Doctor–Patient Relationship in Simone de Beauvoir's *A Very Easy Death*', *Literature and Medicine*, 37.2 (2019), 420–41 (pp. 420–1).

[33] Steven Wilson, *The Language of Disease: Writing Syphilis in Nineteenth-Century France* (Cambridge: Legenda, 2020), p. 8.

medicine in the French nineteenth century. As mentioned previously, nineteenth-century medicine witnessed a progression from eighteenth-century bedside-based medicine to nineteenth-century clinical medicine, and finally to laboratory-based medicine in the twentieth century, propelled by the development of microbiology in the 1850s.[34] Yet the bedside encounter between doctor and patient endures in the cultural imagination. For example, in his autobiography, Lewis Thomas recounts memories of how his physician-father would tend to patients at their own bedside during the first half of the twentieth century.[35] Atul Gawande argues that the shift from bedside to hospital-based medicine was solidified in the middle of the twentieth century, and argues that medicine should return to its previous emphasis on the bedside to provide the compassionate and rational care patients require.[36] Similarly, the bedside is a key literary setting where the contrast between doctor–patient relationship and encounter is played out. Time and again, we see doctors rushing to a patient's bedside and thus being present at a critical moment in a character's, or plot's, development. By examining the cleavage between the idealized doctor–patient relationship and the unpredictable, often disappointing, bedside encounter, nineteenth-century novels challenge the idea of an all-powerful medical hegemony and illustrate it as a negotiation between physician and patient. The dissonance between these two concepts allows novelists to ventriloquize both medical discourse and patienthood, putting them in the service of plot and characterization, and thus produce both elaborate idealizations and criticisms of medicine. The doctor–patient relationship, and the bedside doctor–patient encounter, are therefore crucial ways to illuminate how medicine was understood by, and embedded in, the nineteenth-century novel.

During the first wave of the medical humanities, writers often discussed medical practice without reference to either its contemporary context or historical precedence, with the result that these studies often had a tendency towards reduction. The critical medical humanities now aim at asserting the 'critical' value of paying attention to the past, refocusing scholarship onto periods other than the contemporary.[37] Finally, the critical medical humanities seek to broaden its linguistic and cultural range, historically limited to the English-speaking world, in order to create a global medical humanities.[38] By examining how the development of the French novel is revealed, and its plot and metaphors shaped, by interest in medicine, I contribute to this expanding view of what constitutes the medical humanities.

[34] N. D. Jewson, 'The Disappearance of the Sick-Man from Medical Cosmology, 1770–1870', *International Journal of Epidemiology*, 38.3 (2009), 622–33.

[35] Lewis Thomas, *The Youngest Science: Notes of a Medicine-Watcher* (Oxford: Oxford University Press, 1984), p. 10.

[36] Atul Gawande, *Being Mortal: Illness, Medicine and What Matters in the End* (London: Profile Books, 2014), p. 69.

[37] Whitehead and Woods, 'Introduction', p. 7.

[38] Ibid., p. 2.

This study's conceptualizations of the doctor–patient encounter, the use of medical metaphor, and the construction of medical plots in the nineteenth-century French novel contributes to the ongoing task of building a new critical medical humanities by returning to the concept of the doctor–patient relationship.

Medicine and Narrative

With its focus on literary elements such as plot and metaphor, this study aims to continue the long-standing dialogue between literary studies and the medical humanities at the intersection between narrative and medicine. As we have already seen, the medical humanities' focus on the doctor–patient relationship was fuelled by a newfound critical interest in the idea of the patient's story. The field's subsequent interest in recuperating these narratives about illness and experience to improve the medical consultation points towards the indelible connection between medicine and narrative. Eventually, this connection gave rise to the sub-field of narrative medicine. Narrative medicine originated in the early 1970s when American medical schools began teaching literature to medical students alongside their usual curriculum. Literature was taught in the hope that refining future doctors' interpretative skills would improve both their interpersonal and diagnostic skills, and subsequently the quality of the doctor–patient relationship. Gawande claims that such classes help would-be doctors navigate difficult topics that anatomy, physiology, or neuroscience would neglect: 'I learned a lot of things in medical school, but mortality wasn't one of them. [...] The one time I remember discussing mortality was during an hour we spent on *The Death of Ivan Ilyich*.'[39] Narrative medicine is the stories that the patient tells about their illness and the way in which the doctor attempts to interpret that story. As such, the doctor–patient relationship and encounter are the backdrop against which narrative medicine is played out. Kathryn Montgomery Hunter argues that, firstly, medicine's central aim is to relieve suffering and, secondly, that this suffering can only be understood through the patient. She thus foregrounds medicine's rootedness in interpretation:

> Medicine is an interpretative activity, a learned activity that begins with the understanding of the patient and ends in therapeutic action on the patient's behalf. Far from being object, a matter of hard facts, medicine is grounded in subject knowledge—not of the generalized body in textbooks, which is scientific enough—but the physician's understanding of the particular patient.[40]

[39] Gawande, *Being Mortal*, p. 9.

[40] Kathryn Montgomery Hunter, *Doctors' Stories: The Narrative Structure of Medical Knowledge* (Princeton, NJ: Princeton University Press, 1991), p. xx.

In 2006, Rita Charon published *Narrative Medicine: Honoring the Stories of Illness* in which she outlines the relative pertinence of narrative to medical education: 'what medicine lacks today—in singularity, humility, accountability, empathy—can, in part be provided through intensive narrative training'.[41] Charon argues that narrative and medical practice are both 'suffused with attention to life's temporal horizons, with the commitment to describe the singular, with the urge to uncover plot [...], and with an awareness of the intersubjective and ethical nature of healing'.[42] In this way, the medical humanities' emphasis on narrative medicine as an essential component of illness and healing suggests a parallel between medical or illness narratives and literary narratives *about* medicine or illness.

When it comes to approaching illness narratives, or indeed the related but distinct term of narrative medicine, there is thus a critical cleavage between the medical humanities on the one hand, and literary studies on the other.[43] On the one hand, narrative medicine courses informed by this research often lead to high student satisfaction rates and positive learning outcomes for participants, thanks to the emphasis on interpretative rather than diagnostic approaches to the medical consultation.[44] On the other hand, as a sub-field of the medical humanities, narrative medicine largely ignores the limitations of narrative and storytelling that are the bedrock of literary studies. If all illness has a 'plot', as Charon implies, there must be some form of resolution or outcome to an illness—either convalescence or death. This medical teleology neglects how, for many patients, illness is far more protracted and less resolved than this comparison implies. Even more importantly, scholars observe the reluctance of first-wave medical humanities to question the normative and individualist restrictions imposed through narrative.[45] Frank's work is particularly instructive in this case. As part of his wider argument that narrative is fundamental to illness and recovery, he claims that there are three types of illness narrative: restitution stories which 'attempt to outdistance morality by rendering illness transitory'; chaos stories which fragment under the force of the 'undertow of illness and disasters that attend [illness]'; and quest stories that 'meet suffering head on; they accept illness and seek to *use* it' and thereby recover the self from the fragmented experience of

[41] Rita Charon, *Narrative Medicine: Honoring the Stories of Illness* (New York; Oxford: Oxford University Press, 2006), p. vii.

[42] Ibid., p. 39. Billington argues that literary reading is lacking from modern life yet is particularly important to the doctor–patient relationship in particular. See Billington, *Is Literature Healthy?*, p. 10.

[43] Ann Jurecic, *Illness as Narrative* (Pittsburgh, PA: University of Pittsburgh Press, 2012), p. 3.

[44] Christy DiFrances Remein, Ellen Childs, John Carlo Pasco, and others, 'Content and Outcomes of Narrative Medicine Programmes: A Systematic Review of the Literature through 2019', *BMJ Open*, 10.1 (2020), e031568.

[45] William Viney, Felicity Callard, and Angela Woods, 'Critical Medical Humanities: Embracing Entanglement, Taking Risks', *Medical Humanities*, 41.1 (2015), 2–7 (p. 2).

trauma.[46] However, Frank's hierarchy of illness narratives testifies to the often prescriptive and reductive role played by the concept of narrative in the medical humanities. Woods criticizes Frank for his 'assumption of an innate ahistorical narrative identity upon which his work (and indeed virtually all mainstream medical humanities thinking) is based', that results in narrative having a reductive effect that is unquestioned by medical humanities scholars.[47] Indeed, the limitations of applying Frank's model of narrative, based on the assumed authenticity of the narrative being told, to the complexities and vagaries of literary narrative are clear.

Rather than focusing solely on questions of voice and focalization that narrative medicine emphasizes, I wish to foreground the importance of the structure and function of medical plots to the nineteenth-century French novel. Peter Brooks argues that desire is central to the experience of reading and thus to the construction of plot itself: 'We can, then, conceive of the reading of plot as a form of desire that carries us forward, onward, through the text. Narratives both tell of desire—typically present some story of desire—and arouse and make use of desire as dynamic signification.'[48] The entanglement of narrative with desire is perhaps magnified in the case of medical plots: Chapters Two and Three examine medicine's desire for knowledge, as well as its subversion by female patients. But what interests me most about the nature of literary representations of medicine is the way that medicine, its practitioners, and patients, become entrapped in plot. Medical scenes such as the quintessential bedside encounter between doctor and patient are an event in the plot's construction, often pointing towards a moment of crisis in which a character may lose their life and the novel's plot may take a dramatic new turn. Peter Cryle argues that the pathologies of disease, rather than the powerful gaze of the doctor, provided the novel with its narrative force in the nineteenth century, moving from infection to crisis and then to either convalescence or to death.[49] Whereas Cryle suggests that it is disease that shapes this plot, I suggest that it is the portrayal of the medical relationship and encounter themselves that influences and animates plot. The appearance of the doctor at the patient's bedside not only allows the author an opportunity to combine the novel's other discourses with that of medicine, as well as alter the course of the novel's plot, but it signals to the reader that new elements are being added to the text both in terms of discourse and plot.

[46] Frank, *The Wounded Storyteller*, p. 115.

[47] Angela Woods, 'The Limits of Narrative: Provocations for the Medical Humanities', *Medical Humanities*, 37.2 (2011), 73–8 (p. 75).

[48] Peter Brooks, *Reading for the Plot: Design and Intention in Narrative* (Cambridge, MA; London: Harvard University Press, 1992), p. 37.

[49] Peter Cryle, 'Foretelling Pathology: The Poetics of Prognosis', *French Cultural Studies*, 17.1 (2006), 107–22.

Brian Hurwitz and Victoria Bates outline that narrative continues to bring value to the critical medical humanities when its potential for multiplicity and plurality is observed.[50] I believe that turning to plot helps draw attention to these features. Whereas Brooks sees in plot a singular, desire-oriented movement through the text (motivated either by pleasure or the Freudian death drive), I instead emphasize that medical plots are multistranded: in most of the texts that I analyse, the medical plot is a sideshow to other plots, a mini plot built on top of others, or a moment of crisis that brings all the other plots to a temporary halt. Although narrative and plot are no doubt connected, I view plot as more fragmented and thereby less prone to being subsumed into normative or hegemonic structures. An important conceptual tool to help us understand this aspect is the episodic nature of these medical scenes, as well as the tension between the centrality and peripherality of these medical plots. Elsner observes that, contrary to the critical interest in the doctor–patient relationship, these scenes can be few and far between as in Beauvoir's *Une mort très douce*.[51] Indeed, in the novels that this study examines, scenes revolving around medical encounters are peripheral to the main plot of the novel. My interest in this peripherality differs from the definition of plot proposed by Brooks, who proposes a centrality of events which does not always resonate with medical scenes, which often appear as frequently supplementary to a novel's main plot as they do central to its development. This peripherality may take different forms: patient's encounters with doctors may occupy only one scene in a novel; doctors may appear as side characters in novels; the relationship between doctor and patient may appear frequently at the margins of the novel's main plot.

Of course, there are human experiences which exceed the confines of narrative, often relating to suffering, oppression, and trauma, which narrative may reduce and limit thanks to its propulsion towards normativity and teleology.[52] Lawrence Kirmayer draws attention to metaphor's position between embodiment and the overarching structure inherent to narrative, with the result that 'we may create metaphors with that lack the larger temporal structure of narrative but are no less persistent and powerful'.[53] As Wilson notes, it is the relationship between the body and language, both literary and figurative, that is the focus of literary depictions of medicine.[54] In her essay on tuberculosis, Susan Sontag uses

[50] Brian Hurwitz and Victoria Bates, 'The Roots and Ramifications of Narrative in Modern Medicine', in *The Edinburgh Companion to the Critical Medical Humanities*, ed. by Anne Whitehead and Angela Woods (Edinburgh: University of Edinburgh Press, 2016), pp. 559–76.

[51] Elsner, 'Beyond Medical Paternalism', p. 425.

[52] Woods, 'The Limits of Narrative', p. 76.

[53] Laurence J. Kirmayer, 'Broken Narratives: Clinical Encounters and the Poetics of Illness Experience', in *Narrative and the Cultural Construction of Illness and Healing*, ed. by Cheryl Mattingly and Linda C. Garro (Berkeley, CA: University of California Press, 2000), pp. 153–80 (p. 155).

[54] Wilson, *The Language of Disease*, pp. 9–11.

Stendhal's *Armance* to illustrate that tuberculosis is a uniquely literary disease thanks to its ability to generate a chain reaction of metaphoric signification. This aspect, she argues, allows society to interpret the symptoms of tuberculosis as it may interpret a literary text, thereby retroactively associating consumption with the Romantic disposition, most notably *ennui* and the *mal du siècle*.[55] Hannah Thompson demonstrates how conditions as varied as cholera and paralysis may express a female character's rejection of heteronormative and reproductive sexuality.[56] Understanding metaphors of illness elucidates how medicine is more than a reductive or objective medical gaze. These metaphors can be visual, corporeal, or conceptual and may portray symptoms, pain, or even patient's resistance to their doctors.

Corporeal metaphors, and the way that other medical metaphors connect to the body, is a significant preoccupation of the present study.[57] It goes without saying that, in the humanities, the body is widely understood as a site of both significance and signification. Foucault's analysis of the development of the *regard médical* foregrounds the body as medicine's preeminent object of study, knowledge, and control. In nineteenth-century French literature, then, the body generates meaning and as such is intimately tied to language and narrative: a phenomenon that Thompson's analysis of unspeakable bodies in the nineteenth-century novel, Susan Harrow's study of the 'obsessively corporeal' elements of Zola's *Rougon-Macquart* cycle, and Steven Wilson's examination of literary representations of the syphilitic body all point towards.[58] In the present study I focus not on the concept of corporeality or embodied experience itself, but rather how literary depictions of the body are drawn into the nexus of the doctor–patient relationship. I find that metaphor is consistently used to evoke and make visible the stricken body, and that these metaphors can serve as a significant opportunity for patient resistance against a malevolent doctor. Metaphor thus expands our understanding of nineteenth-century French medical narratives and plots by reaffirming the role played by figurative language in articulating the ill body.

The development of literary narrative in the nineteenth century, most notably of realist modes of mimetic representation, is enmeshed with that of medicine in the period. One of the most important developments made by the Paris School was

[55] Susan Sontag, *Illness as Metaphor; and, AIDS and Its Metaphors* (London: Penguin, 1991), pp. 6–7. Ann Jurecic also observes that Sontag implicitly argues against the therapeutic or personal narrative as a way to represent illness. See Jurecic, *Illness as Narrative*, pp. 72–3.

[56] Hannah Thompson, *Taboo: Corporeal Secrets in Nineteenth-Century France* (Oxford: Legenda, 2013), p. 55.

[57] By focusing on corporeal metaphors, rather than corporeal narratives, I move away from Frank who sees narrative as inherently embodied. See Angela Woods, 'Beyond the Wounded Storyteller: Rethinking Narrativity, Illness and Embodied Self-Experience', in *Health, Illness and Disease: Philosophical Essays*, ed. by Havi Carel and Rachel Cooper (London: Routledge, 2013), pp. 113–28 (p. 120).

[58] See Susan Harrow, *Zola, the Body Modern: Pressures and Prospects of Representation* (London: Legenda, 2010), p. 14.

the newfound interest in the ever-smaller units of biological life. If eighteenth-century medicine focused on localized illness and pain by examining afflicted organs, nineteenth-century medics such as Xavier Bichat were increasingly interested in how illness affected patients on the level of cells and tissues. Bichat 'paved the way for a new form of medicine [...] that displaced the more individualistic, patient-centred medicine of the eighteenth century'.[59] It is these developments that underpin Foucault's concept of the nineteenth-century *regard médical*. The medical gaze, which dehumanized the patient's body by rendering it an object for the doctor's observation, deduction and, ultimately, dissection.[60] Observation via the *regard médical* dehumanized the patient's body, preparing it for diagnosis and treatment. Rather than asking 'Qu'avez vous?' ['What do you have'], the doctor would begin his consultation of the patient with 'Où avez-vous mal?' ['Where does it hurt?'].[61] For Foucault the localization of disease on the patient's body alienates their individuality and subjective experience of illness, reduced to symptoms and lesions by the doctor. He writes,

> À partir de là, tout le rapport du signifiant au signifié se redistribue, [...] à tous les niveaux de l'expérience médicale: entre les symptômes qui signifient et la maladie qui est signifiée, entre la description et ce qu'elle décrit, entre l'événement et ce qu'il pronostique, entre la lésion et le mal qu'elle signale.[62]

> From here, the whole relationship of the signifier to the signified is redistributed, [...] at all levels of medical experience: between the symptoms that signify and the disease that is signified, between the description and what it describes, between the event and what it predicts, between the lesion and the disease that it signals.

The perceived readability of symptoms relies on, but also guarantees 'La coïncidence exacte du "corps" de la maladie et du corps de l'homme malade' ['The exact coincidence of the "body" of the disease and the body of the sick man'].[63] The patient 'n'est par rapport à ce dont il souffre qu'un fait extérieur; la lecture médicale ne doit le prendre en considération que pour le mettre entre parenthèses' ['is, in relation to what he suffers, only an external fact; the medical reading only takes them into account in order to put them in brackets'].[64] In order to understand disease, the individuality of the patient must be subtracted by the doctor: 'Qui veut connaître la maladie dont il s'agit doit soustraire l'individu, avec ses qualités

[59] Thomas R. Cole, Nathan S. Carlin, and Ronald A. Carson, *Medical Humanities: An Introduction* (Cambridge: Cambridge University Press, 2017), p. 49.
[60] Foucault, *Naissance de la clinique*, pp. 5–6.
[61] Ibid., p. 17.
[62] Ibid., p. 17.
[63] Ibid., p. 19.
[64] Ibid., p. 26.

singulières' ['Whoever wants to know the disease in question must subtract the individual, with his singular qualities'].[65]

The predominance of mimetic representation in the nineteenth-century novel means that references to medicine and illness in nineteenth-century novels are most often read as what Roland Barthes identified as the text's *effet de réel* ['reality effect'], examples of the nineteenth-century world that attest to the text's authenticity.[66] Jean-Louis Cabanès's work outlines the importance of linking literary genre to medical practice in order to understand how both the body and illness were conceived: arguing that authors such as Flaubert, the Goncourt brothers, and Zola integrated medical discourse into their novels to heighten verisimilitude.[67] Cabanès therefore builds on Foucault when he states that the representation of medicine in nineteenth-century literature was organized around the new science of observation, or rather 'la modification du regard médical à l'extrême fin du XVIIIème siècle et au tout début du XIXème' ['the change in the medical gaze at the very end of the eighteenth and start of the nineteenth century'] that introduced doctors as characters in the nineteenth-century novel.[68] Lawrence Rothfield argues that medical discourse provided authors with blueprints for realist narrative and epistemology, in addition to a model for the professional authority that authors were beginning to covet for themselves: 'Realist novels do more than incorporate culturally received ideas about science (that they were often hostile to)—they deploy coherent scientific vocabularies and authorities as well as methods and the specific problematics that are posed through these vocabularies and authorities'.[69] Rothfield thus advances an analogy between author and clinician, arguing that texts such as Zola's essay 'Le Roman expérimental' attempted to appropriate the medical gaze that was being developed during the century. Realist vision is thus underpinned by the *regard médical*: 'the relation between author and text is modelled on medical precepts, with the author viewing characters and situations as a doctor views patients and cases'.[70] This appropriation was not always flattering: Flaubert relied on tropes of medical vision at the same time that he satirized medicine and its practitioners. Similarly, Mary Donaldson-Evans illustrates how, beneath French writers' adulation medical science, there lay a 'hidden agenda of undermining the medical profession'.[71]

[65] Ibid., p. 34.

[66] Roland Barthes, 'L'Effet de réel', *Communications*, 11.1 (1968), 84–9.

[67] See Jean-Louis Cabanès, *Le Corps et la maladie dans les récits réalistes (1856–1893)*, 2 vols (Paris: Klincksieck, 1991), I, pp. 243–51.

[68] Ibid., p. 21.

[69] Lawrence Rothfield, *Vital Signs: Medical Realism in Nineteenth-Century Fiction* (Princeton, NJ: University of Princeton Press, 1992), p. 10.

[70] Ibid., p. 37.

[71] Mary Donaldson-Evans, *Medical Examinations: Dissecting the Doctor in French Narrative Prose, 1857–1894* (Lincoln, NE: University of Nebraska Press, 2000), pp. 6–8.

Vision is a central component of the medical relationship, but the effect produced by this incorporation of medical discourse via the motif of the medical gaze cannot be restricted to the 'reality effect' described by Barthes and Cabanès, or to the analogous relationship between realist and medical vision proposed by Rothfield. The inclusion of medicine does not necessarily make the text feel more 'real' to the reader, but rather it enriches the fields of discourse on which the novel relies. In this study I demonstrate how the depiction of the doctor–patient relationship is thus a cornerstone in nineteenth-century texts' literary interactions with medicine. Further, we find that there is not always an analogous relationship between medical and realist vision and, if it does persist, this relationship is continuously interrogated and challenged by medical metaphor itself. Nineteenth-century novels thus appeal to vision and visual language to depict the corporeality of medical practice and the embodied experience of illness. Visual metaphors, particularly when paired with the episodic nature of a medical encounter as we see in Chapters Two and Three, thus complement and challenge the overarching structure of both illness and medical narratives as defined by the medical humanities.

Doctors, Patients, and Power

The binary nature of the doctor–patient relationship invariably evokes questions about the nature of asymmetric or hierarchical power dynamics within medicine. Emanuel and Emanuel's four models of the doctor–patient relationship all hinge on the question of whether the doctor should cede power to the patient in terms of giving information and allowing the patient to determine the path of their own treatment.[72] For his part, Foucault's interest in the intersection between medicine and power during the rest of his career, most notably in *Histoire de la sexualité*, only increases the characterization of the doctor–patient relationship as a space in which power relationships are played out. Given Foucault's work on madness and the nineteenth-century development of sexology, the depiction of hysteria in literary, visual, and popular culture has been a key theme in nineteenth-century French studies. One of the first such studies was Georges Didi-Huberman's exploration of the relationship between psychiatry and nineteenth-century aesthetic culture.[73] Since then interest in hysteria has proliferated to the extent that Mark Micale has referred to the emergence of the field of 'new hysteria studies'.[74] Important studies that adopt a Foucauldian-feminist approach towards medicine in the

[72] Emanuel and Emanuel, 'Four Models of the Physician-Patient Relationship'.
[73] See Georges Didi-Huberman, *Invention de l'hystérie: Charcot et l'iconographie photographique de la Salpêtrière* (Paris: Macula, 1982).
[74] See Mark S. Micale, *Approaching Hysteria: Disease and Its Interpretations* (Princeton, NJ: Princeton University Press, 1994), *passim* for this formulation.

nineteenth century include those by Janet Beizer, Jann Matlock, and Michael Finn.[75] Matlock highlights how, for Foucault, transgressions of the social and sexual order demonstrate that transgressors, such as the prostitute and the hysteric, become 'privileged objects of knowledge in her own right', generating a 'great line of attack' against their bodies.[76] Matlock finds that doctors are the aggressors in this paradigm: hysteria was shaped by medical practitioners, in an 'effort to understand and classify bodies'.[77] In these analyses, the relationship between male doctor and female patient can be understood as one of attempted control and subjugation.

For the patient, however, resistance is still possible. Although the doctor may subtract the patient from their illness, this process of abstraction paradoxically establishes the patient's singularity. Foucault conceptualizes how productive resistance can materialize through the recharging of objects, bodies, and concepts with new meanings or through the inversion of tropes. Although the *regard médical* encourages the doctor to remove the patient from his understanding of the disease or illness, it is, paradoxically, also responsible for creating the new categories of symptoms and signs which existed and produced meaning within frameworks of medical signification, drawing out the patient's individuality.[78] To take an example outside medicine that exemplifies the ubiquity of such a power relationship, in *Histoire de la sexualité* Foucault outlines how confession subjects the confessor to a power matrix which dominates them, but also brings about consciousness of their own subjectivity.[79] As David Armstrong reminds us, it is for this reason that *Naissance de la clinique* can also be characterized as viewing the history of medicine from the perspective of the patient, despite the image of the doctor as omniscient and omnipotent that it creates.[80] In this vein, Didi-Huberman observes how, in Parisian hospitals, hysteria patients would make sexually suggestive comments and gestures towards their doctors, turning the Foucauldian *regard médical* back onto their own doctors.[81] Similarly, scholars such as Naomi Schor and Naomi Segal give critical prominence to the body coded as female, transgressive or in some way ill,

[75] Janet L. Beizer, *Ventriloquized Bodies: Narratives of Hysteria in Nineteenth-Century France* (Ithaca, NY: Cornell University Press, 1994); Jann Matlock, *Scenes of Seduction: Prostitution, Hysteria and Reading Difference in Nineteenth-Century France* (New York: Columbia University Press, 1994); Michael R. Finn, 'Doctors, Malady, and Creativity in Rachilde', *Nineteenth-Century French Studies*, 34.1–2 (2005), 121–33. Although nineteenth-century literature focuses on the female hysteric, the male hysteric was also an important aesthetic trope, see Mark S. Micale, *Hysterical Men: The Hidden History of Male Nervous Illness* (Cambridge, MA; London: Harvard University Press, 2008).

[76] Matlock, *Scenes of Seduction*, p. 3.

[77] Ibid., p. 3.

[78] Foucault, *Naissance de la clinique*, pp. 127–53.

[79] Michel Foucault, *Histoire de la sexualité, 4 vols, i: La Volonté de savoir* (Paris: Gallimard, 1994) pp. 69–98. I pursue this analogy between doctors and priests in more detail in Chapters One and Four.

[80] David Armstrong, 'Bodies of Knowledge / Bodies of Power', in *Reassessing Foucault: Power, Medicine, and the Body*, ed. by Colin Jones and Roy Porter (London; New York: Routledge, 1994), pp. 17–27.

[81] Didi-Huberman, *Invention de l'hystérie*, p. 168.

arguing that the female body becomes a site of resistance because of attempt to control it.[82]

Influenced by these studies' interest in gender and power, I tease out the intersection of medicine and literature with gender and mental disability (including how these elements intersect with one another), observing how medical authority can be resisted by both patients and by the text itself. This challenge is itself constructed and supported by the nature of the doctor–patient relationship which is not a binary power structure but is instead fluid, dynamic, and open to subversion and inversion. Furthermore, in Chapters One and Four, I explore how idealization is a primary function of the doctor–patient relationship, and how this depiction of medicine conserves and perpetuates the paternalistic structures of medicine observed by scholars of hysteria. However, whereas most of the studies mentioned previously focused primarily on hysteria, as well as mental illness more generally, the doctor–patient relationship allows readers to perceive how a myriad of different illnesses and diseases function within the nineteenth-century novel.

Medical Texts

This volume does not pretend to be a directory of all the doctor–patient relationships and encounters portrayed in French novels of the nineteenth century. Instead, by analysing key scenes in a handful of prominent works, I aim at inspiring readers to reassess the ways that they approach literary representations of medicine. By focusing on the doctor–patient relationship, I seek to foreground the relational, practical, and experiential dimensions of nineteenth-century medicine. The fluidity of this relationship gives rise both to medicine's idealization and subversion in ways that are particularly pertinent to questions of gender and disability. Throughout, I return to ideas of medical vision, metaphor, and plot in order to illustrate how literary texts depict medicine. I offer a new interpretation of the role of medicine in the nineteenth-century novel that emphasizes its fluidity, dynamism, and multivalency.

Each chapter of this volume focuses on a cluster of novels that contain important medical episodes. Chapter One, 'Failed Ideals: The Country Doctor and His Patients from Balzac to Zola', explores how Balzac's *Le Médecin de campagne* and Zola's *Le Docteur Pascal* both imagine and idealize doctor–patient relationship through their use of the country doctor trope. I contrast these novels to Flaubert's *Madame Bovary*, arguing that the idealist yet conservative social agenda is crucial to the characterization of the country doctor and the idealization of his

[82] Naomi Schor, *Breaking the Chain: Women, Theory, and French Realist Fiction* (New York: Columbia University Press, 1985); Naomi Segal, *The Adulteress's Child: Authorship and Desire in the Nineteenth-Century Novel* (Cambridge, UK; Cambridge, MA, USA: Polity Press, 1992).

relationship with patients. This chapter's approach is inspired by John Berger's contribution to the medical humanities: his formulation of the country doctor figure in his photo-essay from 1967, *A Fortunate Man: The Story of a Country Doctor.* I establish how Balzac's and Zola's novels engage in this process by using the doctor's relationship with his patients as a metaphor for his relationship with the wider rural community, understood as one based on paternal benevolence and charity. These twinned elements, the doctor's relationship with his patients and with the community, contribute to his heroic characterization by the text. However, this idealized character is plagued by both personal and professional failures, appealing to a more critical view of rural medicine. In the case of Balzac, this disillusionment is achieved through the novel's rewriting of Rousseauian *bienfaisance* ['beneficence']; for Zola, it arises from the novel's turn away from the scientific and experimental approach, that the author espoused in 'Le Roman expérimental', and a re-emphasis on the doctor–patient relationship. In both novels, the idealization of the doctor–patient relationship is part of the novel's conservative discourse surrounding the patient's body, notably in relationship to disability and heteronormative sexual reproduction.

In the two proceeding chapters, this idealized doctor–patient relationship comes under more scrutiny. I examine how novels use the doctor–patient encounter to counter the conservative discourse surrounding the doctor–patient relationship in novels such as *Le Médecin de campagne* and *Le Docteur Pascal.* Chapter Two, 'Blood at the Bedside: Subverting the Medical Relationship in Stendhal', illustrates examples of rebellious female patients who escape the clutches of their overbearing doctors during the doctor–patient encounter. I demonstrate how *Lamiel* appropriates the key features of medical discourse surrounding tuberculosis and undermines the authority of medicine and doctors. The potential deviancy and transgressiveness of the female body are both central to the upended doctor–patient relationships. By focusing on Stendhal's female patients, I reveal them to be active performers of disease who engage with the metaphorical potential of disease, rather than passive victims of either an illness or a malevolent doctor. Taken together, these two features mean that the binary and hierarchical nature of the doctor–patient relationship is questioned in Stendhal's œuvre.

Chapter Three, 'Medical Narratives and Diseased Bodies: Troubling Encounters in Sand and Balzac', explores the use of cholera metaphors in Sand's *Lélia*, written during the 1832 cholera pandemic, to resist the doctor's control of the patient's illness narrative. It also shows how, through the doctor–patient encounter, the novel undermines the supposed authority between the *regard médical*, male desire, and the realist gaze, relying on cholera's corporeality and symptomology to allow the female body to resist invasive enquiry. I demonstrate how *Lélia* pastiches Balzacian depictions of medicine, most notably Horace Bianchon's characterization in the bedside encounter scene in *La Peau de chagrin* and the character's description of his female patients in *Autre étude de femme*. I connect these elements to Bianchon's role in *La Muse du département*, throwing light on how that novel both exemplifies and undermines the doctor's narratorial authority and superior sense of visual knowledge, questioning Bianchon's usually scrupulous ethics. I thus suggest that *Lélia* offers a proto-feminist idealistic view of patienthood in response to Balzac's realism and, moreover, her idealism counters the idealization of the doctor–patient relationship examined in Chapter One.

Chapter Four, 'Zola's *Lourdes* and the Mysteriousness of the Doctor–Patient Relationship', examines how *Lourdes* depicts a patient suffering from hysterical paralysis through the frame narrative of a male character, erasing the patient's own experience of the medical encounters that are recounted. I argue that *Lourdes*'s interest in the male perspective on the female body can be attributed to the novel's interest in demonstrating the harmful effects on women's sexual maturity inspired by the revival of the Marian cult in the mid-nineteenth century. The doctor–patient relationship is presented by Zola as a way for the medic to perceive this issue and thus be able to heal an otherwise incurable patient. I connect the novel's interest in hysteria with the development of microbiology, particularly through the metaphors of invisibility and contagion. I argue that the doctor–patient relationship, despite the apparent threat posed by the microbiological turn, is in fact reconfirmed as the bedrock of medical practice thanks to the idealized and imagined authority that it affords the doctor over his patient.

In its overarching conception, this volume argues that the doctor–patient relationship is an important component of how the nineteenth-century novel narrativizes medicine. Complex and potentially threatening, these literary medical relationships negotiate a wide range of questions and themes, comprising the relationships' participants as well as the epistemological, metaphorical, and narratological aesthetics that underpin them. The forthcoming chapters provide examples of how medicine, art, and science come together to form powerful medical encounters which structure nineteenth-century novelistic representations of the doctor–patient relationship. By critically interrogating the quintessential representation of the doctor–patient relationship, I hope to return readers to the patient's bedside and to encourage them to reconsider how this medical episode can be narrativized and theorized.

Chapter One

Failed Ideals: The Country Doctor and His Patients from Balzac to Zola

Introduction

The demands of rural medicine are well known and range from geographic isolation, social deprivation, increased rates of chronic disease, and restricted access to healthcare. In particular, the 'clinical courage' that rural practitioners display when faced with challenging circumstances has received significant critical attention.[1] These rural struggles and the 'clinical courage' of the doctor mean that the country doctor is a ubiquitous figure in French literature, playing a foundational role in the development of the novel: François Tonnellier observes that 'Le médecin de campagne est le personnage fondateur d'un genre littéraire créé au début du XIXe siècle: le roman médical' ['The country doctor is the founding character of a literary genre that was created at the beginning of the nineteenth century: the medical novel'].[2] How is the country doctor's relationship with his patients depicted, and how does this determine the broader portrayal of medicine in the nineteenth-century French novel? To answer this question, I compare Balzac's *Le Médecin de campagne* and Zola's *Le Docteur Pascal*, arguing that both novels characterize their respective eponymous doctors through the doctor–patient relationship, the connection between doctor and wider community, and the subsequent deific aura that this lends to Benassis and Pascal respectively.

The concept of the country doctor as a distinct form of medical vocation and practice is derived from John Berger's photography-essay *A Fortunate Man: The Story of a Country Doctor*, a cornerstone of the medical humanities that continues to shape how the profession sees itself.[3] Berger's essay discusses the life

[1] Jill Konkin et al. name six features of rural practitioners' 'clinical courage', including the drive to support all members of community, the acceptance of uncertainty, and the provision of collegial support to others so that they may continue their work. See Jill Konkin, Laura Grave, Ella Cockburn, and others, 'Exploration of Rural Physicians' Lived Experience of Practising Outside Their Usual Scope of Practice to Provide Access to Essential Medical Care (Clinical Courage): An International Phenomenological Study', *BMJ Open*, 10.8 (2020), e037705.

[2] François Tonnellier, 'Le *Médecin de campagne*, ou l'ambiguïté des symboles', *Les Tribunes de la santé*, 23 (2009), 57–63 (p. 57).

[3] Billington, *Is Literature Healthy?*, p. 57.

The Doctor–Patient Relationship and the Nineteenth-Century French Novel. Sarah Jones, Oxford University Press.
 DOI: 10.1093/oso/9780198893790.003.0002

and professional experience of rural general practitioner Doctor John Sassall, highlighting the failures and successes of his professional and personal life. As Billington remarks, it elucidates the 'role of the doctor in relation to people's buried lives'.[4] Berger highlights the 'special depth and character' of the medical relationship, which he describes as fundamental to understanding both the country doctor and their wider social significance.[5] The doctor–patient relationship is unique thanks to the physical and emotional intimacy that the patient grants the doctor, physical intimacy 'without a sexual basis' and emotional vulnerability with 'a comparative stranger'.[6] By curing, alleviating, or witnessing pain, the doctor cultivates the position of an 'ideal brother' with his patients: this form of medical fraternity is founded on the doctor's ability to recognize his patient's physical pain and emotional life.[7] However, Berger points out the inevitable failure of the country doctor: overburdened with responsibility, he argues, the doctor realizes the asymmetry inherent in the doctor–patient relationship and grows disillusioned with his vocation.[8]

A Fortunate Man intersperses Berger's prose on the medical relationship with John Mohr's black-and-white photographs of Sassall examining his patients in medical encounters, as well as images with a less overtly medical content. Both forms of image can be read as indices of the doctor–patient relationship, drawing attention to the inherent connection between these two terms. Indeed, the slippage between Berger's focus on the doctor–patient relationship and Mohr's documentation of medical encounters points towards how the doctor–patient relationship and encounter are interconnected in *Le Médecin de campagne* and *Le Docteur Pascal*. As we shall see, both novels use doctor–patient encounters that represent the broader medical relationship that each novel takes as it focus. The medical encounter is both symptom and product of the doctor–patient relationship, which itself represents the doctor's more abstract relationship with the wider community. This chapter argues that the medical relationship itself is inherently social: indeed, it underpins and defines an entire host of social relations organized around Benassis and Pascal respectively. Therefore, the inherent flaws of the doctor–patient relationship strain the doctor, the relationship with his patient and his community, and even the idea of a utopian, curing medical practice. *Le Médecin de campagne* and *Le Docteur Pascal* thus elucidate the limitations of the country doctor trope.

[4] Ibid., p. 59.
[5] John Berger, *A Fortunate Man: The Story of a Country Doctor* (Edinburgh: Canongate Canons, 2016), p. 64.
[6] Ibid., p. 64 and p. 68.
[7] Ibid., p. 69.
[8] Ibid., p. 165.

Fortunate Men: Medicine and the Ideal

Critical analyses of country doctors as represented by nineteenth-century French literature have focused on cynical portrayals of such characters, such as Flaubert's Charles Bovary. In her otherwise comprehensive study of medical characters, Mary Donaldson-Evans pays limited attention to what she admits are the unusually flattering portrayals of Benassis and Pascal, the eponymous characters of *Le Medecin de campagne* and *Le Docteur Pascal* respectively.[9] Such characters are considered to be somewhat unrealistic, a break from the literary connection between nineteenth-century scientism and realism. For example, Lilian Furst compares *Le Médecin de campagne* to *Le Docteur Pascal*, pointing towards the medical progress made in the intervening period between each author's eras, thus suggesting that these scientific advances inform the aesthetics of each novel.[10]

Although this connection between realism and scientism no doubt exists, idealism is particularly important when it comes to the country doctor since, as Berger writes, doctors are both motivated by ideals and become idealized figures themselves.[11] The concept of the doctor–patient relationship is itself founded on an idealistic view of the interpersonal dynamic within, and thus the social potential of, medicine.[12] Idealism and the ideal are crucial, although often overlooked, tenants of nineteenth-century French literature. Most nineteenth-century critics were either explicitly idealistic or tried to integrate realism into idealism, the latter of which was generally acknowledged as the higher form.[13] When, in 1876, Albert Millaud said of Zola's *L'Assommoir* that 'Ce n'est pas du réalisme, c'est de la malpropreté; ce n'est plus de la crudité, c'est de la pornographie' ['It is not realism, it is filth; it is no longer impropriety, it is pornography'], he was criticizing Zola's novel for not containing enough of the idealistic elements that helped define realism. Millaud thus examined Zola according to the aesthetic values of realism, which were supposed to focus on the ordinary in order to uplift its readers and inspire social change.[14] Schor revalorizes the significance of idealism in the nineteenth-century novel, arguing that realism and idealism were considered as interdependent entities by contemporary writers: 'Sand's idealism must [...] be understood as a response to what became known as "Balzacian realism"—although Balzac saw realism as a subcategory of idealism'.[15] In this chapter, I demonstrate

[9] Donaldson-Evans, *Medical Examinations*, p. 18.

[10] Lilian R. Furst, 'Realism and Hypertrophy: A Study of Three Medico-Historical "Cases"', *Nineteenth-Century French Studies*, 22.1/2 (1993), 29–47.

[11] Berger, *A Fortunate Man*, p. 165.

[12] *The Lancet*, 'The Doctor–Patient Relationship: Capturing the Ideal', *The Lancet*, 381.9876 (2013), 1432.

[13] Mary Poovey, 'Forgotten Writers, Neglected Histories: Charles Reade and the Nineteenth-Century Transformation of the British Literary Field', *ELH*, 71.2 (2004), 433–53 (p. 443).

[14] Albert Millaud, 'Lettres fantaisistes sur Paris: M. Émile Zola', *Le Figaro*, 1 September 1876, pp. 1–2 (p. 1).

[15] Naomi Schor, *George Sand and Idealism* (New York: Columbia University Press, 1993), p. 47.

the importance of medical and literary idealism to the depiction of the country doctor, arguing that this aesthetic and political approach sets the parameters for the inevitable failure of the medical relationship between country doctor and his patients. Although reading *Le Médecin de campagne* and *Le Docteur Pascal* from the perspective of the country doctor trope draws on the importance of literary idealism, this idealism should not be considered as part of a more progressive agenda as we shall see in Sand's *Lélia*, discussed in Chapter Three. Instead, in both Balzac and Zola, the country doctor is idealized because of his socially conservative outlook, perceived in the novels' respective attitudes towards family life: Balzac's novel sees Doctor Benassis stimulate his village economically by encouraging sexual reproduction; Zola's novel concludes with the image of Doctor Pascal's child embodying a natalist message of renewal and national regeneration. The Balzacian and Zolian country doctors are best understood as figures of nostalgia, restoration, and social preservation, but also of domination.

The medical relationship is, for both texts, seen on both the level of interactions between doctor and patient and between doctor and his community. What Berger identifies as the 'special character and depth of the doctor–patient relationship' is what allows the medical relationship to function as a microcosm for Benassis's and Pascal's position within their locale.[16] These twinned features contribute to the semi-mythical status of Benassis and Pascal within their community, that of an idealized popular hero. This section focuses on three idealized elements that are essential to the country doctor as according to Berger: the doctor–patient relationship, the doctor's relationship to his local community, and the heroism that characterizes his portrayal.

Le Médecin de campagne revolves around the life and work of Benassis, a doctor who moves to a derelict village in Franche-Comté and attempts to rebuild it according to his own social, economic, and political values, all of which are underpinned by his medical profession. *Le Médecin de campagne* is most often read from the perspective of what the reader learns in its final chapters: firstly, that Benassis's dedication to the village is his way to make amends (without resort to suicide or monastic life) for the death of a young woman he had seduced and the son they had together; secondly, that Genestas visits the village because of his desire to cure his adopted son of his mania for masturbation. As Michael Tilby points out, the anecdotal structure of the novel points towards the characters' innermost secrets: 'au lieu de constituer cette structure faible ou décousue que l'on a tendance à reprocher à l'auteur, l'enchevêtrement des multiples anecdotes à partir desquelles *Le Médecin de campagne* est fabriquée crée entre elles des liens qui situent la signification du texte bien au-delà des limites des choses vues' ['instead of constituting this week or loose structure for which the author tends to be reproached, the entanglement of the multiple anecdotes which comprise *Le Médecin de campagne*

[16] Berger, *A Fortunate Man*, p. 64.

creates links between them that situate the meaning of the text well beyond the limit of what is visible']. [17] Beyond the novel's entanglement of multiple characters' anecdotes, the novel's structure can also be interpreted as being composed of a series of scenes in which the reader either watches an interaction between characters, or listens to a long digression from a character. The relationship that Benassis maintains with his patients characterizes him as the quintessential 'good doctor' and sets the paradigms for how he and his medical work are interpreted. The doctor–patient encounter is thus a recurring motif in the novel, since the narration follows Genestas as he accompanies Benassis during his work. As in Berger's essay, these doctor–patient encounters flow into a more abstract discussion of the doctor–patient relationship, reflecting how the former is a necessary constituent part of the latter.

The novel opens with Commandant Genestas's arrival in an unnamed village in the Dauphiné in 1829. Before Genestas properly enters the town, he converses with a local woman who generously fosters three children and is struggling to maintain them on three francs and a pound of soap per month. Surprised at how little maintenance the woman is given for the children, Genestas engages her in conversation. Although not the primary topic of conversation between the soldier and the woman, Benassis's name is omnipresent in their discussion, indicating that Genestas encounters Benassis through the proxy of a villager. First, Genestas's observation that the three children 'doivent vous coûter deux fois plus' ['must cost you twice as much'] than what she is given is a comment already echoed by the mysterious doctor. [18] Then, Genestas discovers that the woman owes money to the local miller, but the miller's connection to Benassis means that the woman is not particularly concerned about her debt: 'Je dois soixante-quinze francs au meunier pour de la farine. Heureusement, c'est le meunier de monsieur Benassis. Monsieur Benassis, voilà un ami du pauvre! Il n'a jamais demandé son dû à qui que ce soit, il ne commencera point par nous' ['I owe the miller seventy-five francs for flour. Fortunately, he's also Monsieur Benassis's miller. Monsieur Benassis, now that is a friend of the poor! He has never asked for his due from anyone, and he will not start with us']. [19]

Finally, Genestas poses the following question: 'Monsieur Benassis est-il un bon médecin?' ['Is Monsieur Benassis a good doctor?']. [20] The woman's response extricates the soldier's insinuation from the ambiguity of the word 'bon' ['good']. She answers: 'Je ne sais pas, mon cher monsieur, mais il guérit les pauvres pour rien' ['I don't know, but he heals the poor for free'], suggesting that although she

[17] Michael Tilby, '*Le Médecin de campagne* et le statut du récit', *L'Année balzacienne*, 4.1 (2003), 7–24 (p. 21).

[18] Honoré de Balzac, *Le Médecin de campagne*, ed. by Jean A. Ducourneau (Paris: Livre de Poche, 1966), p. 21.

[19] Ibid., pp. 22–3.

[20] Ibid., p. 25.

is unsure about how effective Benassis's medical practice may be, his generosity towards the poor demonstrates that he is *bon* in the moral sense of the word.[21] The trope of not charging the poor is repeated merely a few pages later, Benassis tells Genestas that he only needs to repay the doctor for his own bed and board if he is wealthy, 'Si vous êtes riche [...] vous paierez bien, sinon, je ne veux rien' ['If you are rich you will certainly pay, if not, I will charge you nothing'], both confirming Benassis's philanthropy and suggesting that Genestas and Benassis have already entered into a form of the doctor–patient relationship.[22] The country doctor's philanthropism is confirmed by Berger as an integral part of his identity and relationship to his patients: 'a doctor who has surpassed the stage of selling cures [...] is unassessable'.[23] Even before Benassis is properly introduced, he is represented through the frame of his relationship with patients: he is generous, invested in their everyday lives, and protects their interests in the wider community. The particularity of the country doctor's relationship with his patients is thus anticipated by Genestas's encounter with a villager, which acts as a proxy for Genestas's own encounter with the doctor.

In the Introduction of the present study, I commented on the slipperiness between the doctor–patient relationship and encounter. In *Le Médecin de campagne*, this slippage between the medical encounter and relationship is exploited: a doctor–patient encounter, witnessed by Genestas, is used metonymically to stand in for the medical relationship that Benassis shares with his patients. A few pages after encountering the villager, Genesta eventually meets Benassis and accompanies him on an urgent house visit during which the doctor tends to the bedside of a dying patient, a likely sufferer from what is now understood to be congenital iodine deficiency syndrome that can impair mental and physical development. The novel portrays Benassis as a paternalistic, benevolent caregiver, but this position is largely based on the narrator's self-proclaimed disgust at the patient and his way of life, thereby characterizing as possessing almost superhuman compassion due to his sympathetic treatment of a person whom the narrator regards as subhuman. Here *Le Médecin de campagne* departs from one key element of Berger's concept, that the doctor should treat the patient 'as a total personality'.[24] The narrator describes the so-called horror of encountering a sufferer of this congenital disease for the first time:

> Malgré les innombrables spectacles de sa vie militaire, le vieux cavalier ressentit un mouvement de surprise accompagné d'horreur en apercevant une face humaine où la pensée ne devait jamais avoir brillé, face livide où la souffrance

[21] Ibid., p. 25.
[22] Ibid., p. 50.
[23] Berger, *A Fortunate Man*, p. 167.
[24] Ibid., p. 62.

apparaissait naïve et silencieuse, comme sur le visage d'un enfant qui ne sait pas encore parler et qui ne peut plus crier, enfin la face toute animale d'un vieux crétin mourant.[25]

Despite the innumerable spectacles of his military life, the old cavalryman felt a movement of surprise accompanied by horror when he perceived a human face where thought must never have shone, a deathly pale face where suffering appeared naïve and silent, like the face of a child who does not yet know how to speak and who can no longer cry, certainly the entirely animal face of a dying old cretin.

Relying on ableist discourse that styles the physically and mentally disabled patient as a minor, or even an animal, this passage uses Genestas's military background to foreground the supposed horror of confronting the patient. Also notable is how the word 'crétin' is used instead of 'malade' or 'homme', underlining what the narrator perceives as the sub-human status of the patient.

Although Genestas finds it difficult to 'lui accorder un regret' ['grant him any sympathy'] because of what he identifies as the pitifulness of his existence, the scene becomes more sympathetic to the patient. Benassis's dedication to his patient is demonstrated through his use of touch, which appears unflinchingly brave in contrast to Genestas's recoil at the sight of the patient: 'Benassis lui-même, après avoir étudié cette face morte et ces yeux sans lumière, vint prendre doucement la main du crétin et lui tâta le pouls' ['Benassis, after having studied that dead face and those lightless eyes, came gently to take the cretin's hand and felt his pulse'].[26] Benassis then declares that the bath is not doing the patient any good, lifts him from it, and carries him to what will become his deathbed:

Il prit lui-même cette masse de chair, la transporta sur le grabat d'où il venait sans doute de la tirer, l'y étendit soigneusement en allongeant les jambes déjà presque froides, en plaçant la main et la tête avec les attentions que pourrait avoir une mère pour un enfant.[27]

He took this mass of flesh, carried him to the pallet from which he had no doubt just lifted him, and carefully laid him on it by stretching out his legs, which were already almost cold, arranging his hands and head with the attention that a mother would have had for her child.

This passage sees the patient dehumanized, reduced to a mound of flesh. By objectifying the patient, and emphasizing his weight, his 'masse de chair', the passage

[25] Balzac, *Le Médecin de campagne*, p. 37.
[26] Ibid, p. 38.
[27] Ibid, p. 38.

foregrounds Benassis's superior physical strength by commenting that he lifts him up 'lui-même'. This display of masculine strength is set into relief by his tenderness. Benassis moves the patient back to the rudimentary bed from which the narrator speculates he has just carried him; the doctor 'soigneusement' moves the patient's limbs. Further, the quasi-maternal aspects of the doctor–patient relationship are made evident: the doctor arranges the patient on the bed 'avec les attentions que pourrait avoir une mère pour un enfant'. As Benassis foresaw, the patient dies only a few moments later. The opening of *Le Médecin de campagne* thus offers a grim portrayal of the country doctor's daily rounds, yet Benassis's encounter with his patient offers a single ray of hope amidst this picture. Here the doctor–patient encounter is elided with the medical relationship: as a naïve onlooker, Genestas uses this single encounter to deduce the nature of Benassis's more general, and more abstract, medical relationship with his other patients. At the same time, the relationship between the country doctor and his patients is presented as a way that Genestas can understand, perhaps even diagnose, the character and values of Benassis, although at the cost of the dehumanization of the patient.

Berger argues that the country doctor is both embedded in the local community and the moral leader of it, a feature of medical paternalism that is inaugurated and anticipated by the doctor–patient relationship.[28] The doctor's relationship to his community is also emphasized by Balzac's novel, particularly since this form of ethical leadership is seen as the panacea for 'le grand malade social' ['huge social illness'] that he perceived as haunting France after the 1789 Revolution.[29] The patient's death itself inspires Benassis, in an extended monologue, to recount his arrival at what was at the time an isolated village. Here the novel harks back to the values perceived to have been destroyed by the Revolution, since the action takes place in an area of France entirely dislocated from contemporary political events: 'Aucun événement politique, aucune révolution n'était arrivée dans ce pays inaccessible, et complètement en dehors du mouvement social' ['No political event, no revolution had happened in this land that was both inaccessible and completely outside national social life'].[30] However, this section of the novel is not just a 'tedious exposition of Balzac's ideas on political economy' as William Paulson suggests.[31] Instead, Benassis's monologue builds on the doctor–patient encounter that precedes it and, in turn, folds out onto a more abstract conception of the medical relationship that Benassis maintains with his villagers.

Given the impoverished state of the village and its community, Benassis resolves to improve the health of the village as well as that of his patients, 'Je voulus

[28] Berger, *A Fortunate Man*, p. 111

[29] See José-Luis Diaz, 'Balzac romancier de la "grande maladie sociale" (1838–1847)', *L'Année balzacienne*, 17.1 (2016), 221–40.

[30] Balzac, *Le Médecin de campagne*, p. 60.

[31] William Paulson, 'Preceptors, Fathers, and Ideology: The Strange Narrative of Balzac's *Le Médecin de campagne*', *French Forum*, 9.1 (1984), 19–32 (p. 20).

devenir l'ami des pauvres sans attendre d'eux la moindre récompense' ['I wanted to become a friend of the poor without expecting anything whatsoever in return from them'].[32] Benassis social cure for the *bourg* is to spark economic industriousness. Benassis explains that installing a basket-maker was fundamental to transforming the local economy since, inspired by the basket-maker's entrepreneurship, a road soon followed, allowing goods to flow more easily to market, and so the road was 'la cause la plus directe de la prospérité future du bourg' ['the most direct route towards the village's future prosperity'].[33] The town now produces wine, a symbol of the town's newfound fecundity: 'Le vin, jadis inconnu dans le bourg, où l'on ne buvait que des piquettes, y devint naturellement un besoin' ['Wine, previously unknown in the village, where only poor imitations were drunk, naturally became a necessity there'].[34] Increased economic productivity was channelled by Benassis into sexual reproduction and domestic harmony: the doctor orchestrates the basketmaker's marriage to a local woman in order to shape the habits of the other villagers by setting them an example to follow. In this way, Benassis's political agenda is influenced by ethical and moral considerations, rather than self-promotion.[35]

Despite his efforts to improve the village, Benassis rejects Genestas's suggestion that he should consider running for government. As Elisabeth Gerwin persuasively argues, this form of political leadership would reward Benassis more than the people he represents, and thus would embody 'le mal du narcissime' that Benassis rails against elsewhere in the novel.[36] According to Benassis, he has merely performed the duty required of a country doctor who must act as a kind of magistrate insofar as he is responsible for the health of both his patients and the wider community.[37] The idea of the doctor-as-magistrate has significant precedence, most notably in the priestly father figure of the *médecin-philosophe*, a trope which persisted throughout the nineteenth century.[38] Indeed Pierre-Jean-Georges Cabanis wrote that: 'Sous certains rapports, la profession de médecin est une espèce de sacerdoce: sous d'autres, c'est une véritable magistrature' ['In some respects, the medical profession is a kind of priesthood: in other respects it is a real magistracy'].[39] For Cabanis, the doctor's role as a magistrate over his patients

[32] Balzac, *Le Médecin de campagne*, p. 61.
[33] Ibid., p. 67.
[34] Ibid., pp. 75–6.
[35] For a similar argument, see Max Andréoli, 'Morale de la politique et politique de la morale dans *La Comédie humaine*', *L'Année balzacienne*, 4.1 (2003), 125–60.
[36] Elisabeth Gerwin, 'Le Mal du narcissisme chez Balzac', *L'Année balzacienne*, 17.1 (2016), 325–42.
[37] Balzac, *Le Médecin de campagne*, p. 86.
[38] For the appearance of this trope in Proust, see Elsner, 'À la recherche du médecin-philosophe'.
[39] Pierre-Jean-Georges Cabanis, *Du Degré de certitude de la médecine* (Paris: Crapat & Ravier, 1803), p. 151. The doctor's medical magistracy forms the basis of Flaubert's criticism of the idealized *médecin de campagne*. In a letter to George Sand dated 1873, Flaubert wrote: '*Les médecins devraient être des magistrats*, afin qu'ils puissent forcer ..., etc' ['*Doctors should be magistrates*, so that they can force .... etc.']. Letter to George Sand of 3 February 1873, in Gustave Flaubert, *Correspondance*, ed. by Jean

is derived from the necessity to heal rather than merely to prescribe medication: 'C'est peu qu'il sache médicamenter; il faut qu'il sache guérir' ['It would not be enough to know how to medicate; he has to know how to heal'].[40] To do this, the doctor 'n'a pas moins besoin de connaître les divers effets des impressions morales, que ceux des remèdes ou des aliments: il faut qu'il soit initié dans tous les secrets du cœur, qu'il sache en remuer à propos toutes les fibres sensibles' ['does not have less need to know the various effects of moral impressions than those of remedies or food: he must be initiated into all the secrets of the heart, know how to stir all the body's sensitive fibres appropriately'].[41]

The doctor should expand his medical role to include that of the magistrate, entailing an exercise of the law and the control of transgressive individuals to heal the body politic. Cabanis thus creates an analogy between the doctor's medical control of the individual's body which could be projected onto the legal control of the civil body, thereby insinuating that the doctor–patient relationship becomes the key site where the doctor's authority over the individual translates into civic power. In this way, the doctor's relationship with his patients, and particularly his dominance over and superiority to them, serves as a mandate for control over the public body as well as that of his patient.

In contrast to adopting his quasi-magistrate's, role, seeking political office would be tantamount to succumbing to what Benassis characterizes as the disease of the century, man's desire to set himself apart from others, 'La maladie de notre temps est la superiorité' ['The illness of our time is superiority'].[42] Benassis instead sees his medical profession as part of the professional triad of *robes noires*: priests, lawyers, and doctors, whose work seeks to protect the conscience, property, and health of their community. In order to increase production and continue to civilize the locale, Benassis argues that the benevolent authority of the *robes noires* must be recognized by the local people, and that the professionals themselves should also assume the burden of preserving and improving their clients and their community. He says:

> Pour civiliser, pour créer des productions, il faut faire comprendre aux masses en quoi l'intérêt particulier s'accorde avec les intérêts nationaux qui se résolvent par les faits, les intérêts et les principes. Ces trois professions, en touchant nécessairement à ces résultats humains, m'ont donc semblé devoir être aujourd'hui les plus grands leviers de la civilisation; ils peuvent seuls offrir

Bruneau, 5 vols (Paris: Gallimard, 1973–2007), IV, 642. For Stendhal's criticism of the analogy drawn between doctor, priest, and magistrate, see Francesco Manzini, 'Doctors, Priests, Magistrates: Stendhal, Cabanis and the Power of Medical Practitioners', in *Institutions and Power in Nineteenth-Century French Literature and Culture*, ed. by David Evans and Kate Griffiths (Leiden: Brill, 2011), pp. 167–82.

[40] See Cabanis, *Du Degré de certitude*, p. 152.

[41] Ibid., pp. 152–3.

[42] Balzac, *Le Médecin de campagne*, p. 88.

constamment à un homme de bien des moyens efficaces d'améliorer le sort des classes pauvres, avec lesquelles ils ont des rapports perpétuels.[43]

In order to civilize, in order to generate production, it is necessary to make the masses understand how particular interests accord with national interests which are resolved by facts, interests, and principles. These three professions, necessarily affecting these human results, therefore seem to me to be today the greatest facilitators of civilisation; they alone can constantly offer man a more effective means of improving the lot of the poorer classes, with whom they have a perpetual relationship.

This passage's insistence on the word 'rapport' indicates that the doctor's relationship with his community is based on, and indeed composed of, relationships and encounters between himself and his individual patients. The doctor's interpersonal relationship with patients, the mix of heroism and tenderness witnessed in the novel's opening medical scene, is the model through which the doctor heals his community by improving the village's sanitation infrastructure that is itself funded by the economic and sexual productivity that the doctor encourages. Benassis's quasi-paternal relationship to both his individual patients and to the wider community means that he feels secure in the local vicinity, as he tells Genestas: 'L'affection tacite des habitants est tout ce que j'ai personnellement gagné à ces changements, outre le plaisir de m'entendre dire par tout le monde d'un air joyeux, quand je passe: Bonjour, Monsieur Benassis!' ['The tacit affection of the inhabitants is all that I have personally gained from these changes, beside the pleasure of hearing the pleasure of everyone saying cheerfully when I pass by: Hello, Monsieur Benassis!'].[44] But, as we shall see in the second half of this chapter, the doctor's assertion that the community wholeheartedly welcomes him is disrupted later in the novel and the hierarchy of the paternal doctor–patient relationship is thus questioned on a textual level.

Zola's novel also hinges on the metonymic relationship between the country doctor's relationship with his patients, itself portrayed through singular encounters, and his wider community. *Le Docteur Pascal* focuses on the life and death of the eponymous doctor, who lives with his niece Clotilde and his mother Félicité, and eventually enters a romantic relationship with the former. The novel traces Pascal's main medical interests, the famous *arbre généalogique* [genealogical tree] and his experimental injection therapy, contributing to the critical characterization of Zola as a scientific author. In 'Le Roman expérimental' Zola famously contends that there exists an analogy between literature and science, arguing that

[43] Ibid., p. 95.
[44] Ibid., p. 84.

literature should adopt the experimental method Doctor Claude Bernard was contemporaneously applying to medicine. Zola ostensibly adopts a doctrine of determinism: 'les lois de la pensée et des passions seront formulées à leur tour. Un même déterminisme doit régir la pierre des chemins et le cerveau de l'homme' ['The laws of thought and passion will be formulated in turn. The same determinism must rule the stone of the paths and of the human brain'].[45] Zola sees the scientist and writer as united in their search for 'le mécanisme' ['the mechanism'] that animates life; the writer's literary experiment is to imagine certain conditions, and then write what they observe.[46] This analogy between doctor and writer has generated significant critical interest in the overlap between medicine and the Naturalist novel. Lawrence Rothfield argues that the nineteenth-century novel adopted the *regard médical* as part of the development of realism as well as the professionalization of writing.[47] David Baguley also observes the extent to which scientific ideas pervaded Zola's work, despite the clumsy inclusion of the spontaneous combustion of Antoine Macquart.[48]

However, *Le Docteur Pascal* can also be understood from the perspective of the literary trope of the country doctor, since the novel focuses on the doctor's relationship with his patients as well as his status in, and his relationship with, the local community. My argument here builds on observations made by Andrew Counter and Claire White regarding Zola's move towards idealism and utopianism from 1894 onwards, and I advance that idealism shapes *Le Docteur Pascal* as much as it does in later works such as *Lourdes*.[49] The latter novel engages with the idealization of the country doctor from the beginning of the novel. Zola's novel opens with the image of Pascal sequestered in his study, surrounded by a library of books that he uses for his medical research. In the final section of this chapter, I suggest how this image of a *médecin-expérimentateur* ['doctor-experimenter'] is almost immediately disrupted; but here I would like to focus on how the second chapter moves the novel from Pascal's study and focuses on his itinerant medical practice in the local community. Although Pascal may be best known as the scientist of the *Rougon-Macquart*, I argue that the novel thus establishes him as a country doctor through, firstly, the depth and character of the doctor–patient relationships he forms and, secondly, the connection his community that originates within his medical relationships.

[45] Émile Zola, *Le Roman expérimental*, ed. by François-Marie Mourad (Paris: Flammarion, 2006), p. 59.

[46] Ibid., p. 56.

[47] See Rothfield, *Vital Signs*.

[48] David Baguley, *Naturalist Fiction: The Entropic Vision* (Cambridge: Cambridge University Press, 1990), p. 63.

[49] Andrew J. Counter, 'Zola's *fin-de-siècle* Reproductive Politics', *French Studies*, 68.2 (2014), 193–208; Claire White, 'Labour of Love: George Sand's *La Ville noire* and Émile Zola's *Travail*', *The Modern Language Review*, 106.3 (2011), 697–708.

In *Le Médecin de campagne*, Benassis's medical rounds are a central motif of the country doctor trope insofar as they allow the narration to focus on the 'doctor in the field', testing his practical skills and bedside demeanour. *Le Docteur Pascal* contains a similar scene that uses the doctor–patient relationship to reveal the nature of Pascal's medical and professional life. Although Pascal is mostly retired from active practice in *Le Docteur Pascal*, chapter two takes place on a Thursday, Pascal's 'jour de visites' ['visiting day'].[50] Pascal invites Clotilde on his rounds, who is the main narrative focalizer of the scene. The pair walk into Plassans and happen to cross paths with Doctor Ramond, a much younger doctor who is setting up a practice in the town. Ramond asks Pascal for his most recent research on consumption, and they converse with one another: Ramond 'écoutait avec déférence le docteur Pascal, dont il admirait beaucoup les travaux' ['listened deferentially to Doctor Pascal, whose work he greatly admired'].[51] Seen through Clotilde's eyes, this encounter between colleagues characterizes Pascal as a patriarch of the local medical establishment. Pascal explains to Ramond that he and Clotilde are on their way to the home of Guiraude. Pascal briefly recounts to Ramond the medical history of the family: the father died five years ago from tuberculosis and was survived by a wife and two children. Pascal proudly informs Ramond that both the children have survived, proving correct his suspicions that consumption was not a hereditary disease: 'voyez si j'ai raison de prétendre que la phtisie n'est pas héréditaire, mais que les parents phtisiques lèguent seulement un terrain dégéneré, dans lequel la maladie se développe, à la moindre contagion' ['see if I am correct in claiming that consumption is not hereditary, but that consumptive parents bequeath only a degenerated ground in which the disease develops as a result of the slightest contagion'].[52] Pascal points to the respective fates of the children to prove his point: 'Valentin, qui a vécu dans le contact quotidien du père, est phtisique, tandis que Sophie, poussée en plein soleil, a une santé superbe' ['Valentin, who has lived in daily contact with his father, is consumptive; whereas Sophie, who grew up in the sun, is in superb health'].[53]

Zola here incorporates into the text relatively new scientific knowledge about tuberculosis in order to 'prove' the accuracy of Pascal's theory, although not so novel that readers would not readily have understood it.[54] Earlier in the century tuberculosis was primarily understood to be caused by hereditary factors, and was only conclusively proven to be contagious in 1869 by Jean Antoine Villemin.[55]

[50] Émile Zola, *Le Docteur Pascal*, ed. by Henri Mitterand (Paris: Gallimard, 2017), p. 98.
[51] Ibid., p. 100.
[52] Ibid., p. 101.
[53] Ibid., p. 101.
[54] I borrow the word 'incorporation' from Larry Duffy's analysis of the scientific hypotheses on which vraisemblance in *Le Docteur Pascal* relies. See Duffy, *Flaubert, Zola*, pp. 194–217.
[55] For an excellent overview of René Laënnec's revolutionary approach to consumption, as it was then known, see Jacalyn Duffin, *To See with a Better Eye: A Life of R. T. H. Laennec* (Princeton, NJ; Chichester: Princeton University Press, 1998).

In *Le Docteur Pascal*, the doctor points out that the disease is spread through contagion and close contact, a fact that would have been widely known in the 1890s when the novel was published, but, in 1872 when the novel takes place, this fact had only been established for three years. The chronology of advances in the understanding of tuberculosis thus allows Zola to characterize Pascal as in touch with the science of medicine, particularly in comparison to Ramond who is revealed to still naively believe in outdated hereditary theory. In this scene, then, Pascal is represented as primordially interested in the science of medicine: in the subsequent pages, however, frame him as equally entangled in the intricacies of the doctor–patient relationship and his connection to Plassans.

Pascal and Clotilde eventually arrive at Guiraude's family home, finding a scene of destitution as the doctor had warned. Berger also points out the proximity of the country doctor to rural poverty, and thus the doctor's task to recognize that some illness are caused by societal or environmental conditions.[56] Guiraude is described as thin and overworked yet thrilled to see Pascal: '[elle] sourit pourtant, ce jour là, en apercevant le docteur, car Valentin venait de manger une côtelette, de grand appétit, véritable débauche qu'il ne se permettait pas depuis des mois' ['However, [she] smiled that day when she saw the doctor because Valentin had just eaten a chop with great appetite, a real feast which he had not allowed himself for months'].[57] The text suggests that Valentin's renewed strength is due to Pascal's seemingly miraculous injections: earlier Pascal tells Ramond that 'je vais peut-être sauver Valentin, car il renaît à vue d'œil, il engraisse, depuis que je le pique' ['I might be able to save Valentin, since he looks like a new person, he's gaining weight ever since I've been injecting him']; when they get to Guiraude's home, '[Valentin] s'était [...] levé avec promptitude, pour montrer qu'il était gaillard' ['[Valentin] stood up quickly, to show that he was a strapping young lad'].[58] Susan Harrow points out that Pascal's project of repairing defective cells or tissue through the introduction of healthy cells anticipates modern-day serum therapy, suggesting that his 'scientific passion, harnessed to a humanitarian, utopian idea, envisions a future of perfection and happiness, with sound health for all'.[59] By describing Valentin's physical appearance, the novel provides seemingly undeniable evidence that Pascal's interventions are improving the patient's condition.

The doctor–patient relationship is, in this scene, particularly emotionally charged. Seen through Clotilde's eyes, the text describes how:

> Aussi Clotilde fut-elle émue de l'acceuil fait à Pascal, comme au sauveur, au messie attendu. Ces pauvres gens lui serraient les mains, lui auraient baisé les pieds, le regardaient avec des yeux luisants de gratitude. Il pouvait donc tout, il était donc

[56] Berger, *A Fortunate Man*, p. 74.
[57] Zola, *Le Docteur Pascal*, pp. 101–2.
[58] Ibid., pp. 101, 102.
[59] Harrow, *Zola, the Body Modern*, p. 39, n. 40.

> le bon Dieu. [...] Il le piqua [Valentin] de nouveau, pendant que Clotilde, debout devant la fenêtre, tournait le dos; et, lorsqu'ils partirent, elle le vit qui laissait vingt francs sur la table. Souvent, cela lui arrivait, de payer ses malades, au lieu d'en être payé.[60]
>
> So moved was Clotilde by the welcome given to Pascal, like that given to the saviour, the awaited messiah. These poor people shook his hand, would have kissed his feet, looked at him with eyes shining with gratitude. He could do anything; he was the good Lord. [...] He injected [Valentin] again while Clotilde, standing in front of the window, turned her back; and when they left she saw him leaving twenty francs on the table. Often this happened, paying his patients instead of being paid for his services.

Relying on free indirect discourse, this passage begins by describing Clotilde's emotional response to Pascal's welcome at the house before moving into her impression of the scene, which is inevitably framed by a semantic field of religion reflecting her devotion to Catholicism ('sauveur', 'messie', 'le bon Dieu', 'ressuscitait les morts'). The gratitude towards Pascal is also seen through Clotilde's framework of Christian motifs: the change to the conditional perfect ('auraient baisé les pieds') from the imperfect ('serraient les mains') indicates a shift between Clotilde's observation of the scene and her speculation about the more symbolic meaning of what is happening. The passage's focalization then zooms back out to describe Clotilde standing at the window, detailing that she sees him leave money for the family. The narrator then adds a new detail that Clotilde probably could not know, since she rarely accompanies Pascal's on his rounds, namely that the doctor donates money more often than he receives it. In this scene, the relationship between Valentin and his mother is the vehicle for what Harrow characterizes as Pascal's idealistic approach to medicine.

After visiting three other patients, Pascal and Clotilde walk to Séguiranne in order to see Sophie, Valentin's healthy sister who lives with their aunt. In comparison to Guiraude's home, Séguiranne is a lush oasis: 'Les platanes, les marroniers, les ormeaux poussaient vigoureusement' ['Plane trees, chestnuts, elms all grew vigorously'].[61] Befitting to her surroundings, and as Pascal suggested earlier, Sophie is a beacon of health. The text remarks on how her previously gaunt features, her 'petite taille, ses pommettes saillantes, ses cheveux pâles' ['small build, her protruding cheekbones, her light hair'], have been improved by her new life. The narrator details that 'à la campagne, loin de la contagion du milieu paternel, il semblait qu'elle eût pris de la chair, d'aplomb sur ses fortes jambes, les joues remplies, les cheveux abondants' ['in the countryside, far from the contagion of the familial

[60] Zola, *Le Docteur Pascal*, p. 102.
[61] Ibid., p. 103.

home, she seemed to have filled out, her strong legs had grown, her cheeks had filled out, and her hair had become thicker'].[62] The narrator links her good health (and beauty) to gratitude, remarking that 'elle avait de très beaux yeux, qui luisaient de santé et de gratitude' ['she had very beautiful eyes, which shone with health and gratitude'].[63] Since Sophie is not ill, she is not Pascal's patient (her aunt remarks 'Ah! Monsieur Pascal, nous n'avons pas besoin de vous, ici! il n'y personne de malade!' ['Oh, Monsieur Pascal, we don't need you here! There's no one ill here!']): nevertheless she is deeply grateful for the doctor's services, suggesting that Pascal's connection to her extends beyond the conventional doctor–patient relationship. Her thankfulness is both in response to Pascal preventing her from becoming like her brother, and the work that Pascal does in order to try to save him.

For all Pascal's dedication to science, he is nonetheless embedded in the local community via his relationships with patients and their families. Unlike *Le Médecin de campagne*, though, *Le Docteur Pascal* does not suggest that the eponymous doctor healed or significantly improved the local town. Rather than the focus on community that we see in *Le Médecin de campagne*, Le *Docteur Pascal* focuses primarily on the theme of family, both Pascal's immediate family and his tracing of the family tree. As we shall soon see, the novel also revolves around the natalist message of Pascal's eventual embrace of 'life' through sexual procreation, that is to say, through the perpetuation of the family. By contrast, Benassis's confession reveals that he has decided to put his energy into saving the village after his attempts to create and support a family collapsed. In *Le Médecin de campagne*, the country doctor's relationship to the community is not just modelled on the doctor–patient relationship, but also serves as a replacement for the doctor's own family. In this dual way, split between family and community, the country doctor in both Balzac and Zola is seen to be indelibly rooted in their wider social space.

A feature of *Le Docteur Pascal* that is particularly striking is the extent to which Pascal is seen as a God-like figure by his patients and the wider community, coinciding with how Berger observes that the doctor is a 'popular hero' and the 'most idealized of the professions'.[64] As mentioned previously, the scene at Guiraude's house demonstrates the reverence with which the locals treat the doctor. Here Pascal's ability to improve the health of patients who are otherwise doomed gives him the power of resurrection and thus a God-like status. Note that this passage is focalized through Clotilde, who sees Pascal's medical experiments as miracles

[62] Ibid., p. 104. The importance of labour is also highlighted in this passage: Sophie and her aunt work in abundant fields; whereas Valentin is reliant on his mother shelling almonds to make an income for the pair. *Le Docteur Pascal* thus echoes the emphasis in *Le Médecin de campagne* on the link between economic prosperity and health.

[63] Zola, *Le Docteur Pascal*, p. 104.

[64] Berger, *A Fortunate Man*, p. 165. For a short study on the idealization of doctors in an American context, see Evelyn Wilbanks, 'The Doctor as Romantic Hero: A Study of Idealization', *JAMA*, 220.1 (1972), 54–7.

condoned by God. Later in the novel the narrator notes 'Elle restait, au fond, la fervente du mystère; et elle disait gaiement que, [si Pascal] faisait ainsi des miracles, c'était qu'il en avait en lui le pouvoir, un vrai bon Dieu!' ['She remained, deep down, a fervent believer; and she said happily that, [if Pascal] performs miracles like this, it was because he had the power within him, and was truly a good Lord'].[65] That Clotilde is characterized as a 'fervente du mystère' throws light on what the text portrays as her naïve religious beliefs: at this point in the novel, before her conversion to Pascal's experimental method, she can only understand the doctor's medical practice through the paradigm of religion.

The narration itself favours a semantic field of sovereignty and kingship to describe Pascal in more secular terms. As Pascal and Clotilde walk through Plassans on their way to Guiraude's house, the doctor is described as an ancient king: 'On aurait dit un de ces anciens rois qu'on voit dans les tableaux, un de ces rois puissants et doux qui ne vieillissent plus, la main posée sur l'épaule d'une enfant belle comme le jour, dont la jeunesse éclatante et soumise les soutient' ['He looked like one of those ancient kings depicted in paintings, like one of those powerful and gentle kings who no longer age, his hand resting on the shoulder of a child as beautiful as the day, whose radiant and submissive youth supports his hand'].[66] Later in the novel, as the romantic relationship between Clotilde and Pascal begins to blossom and the couple seclude themselves in the house, Clotilde completes a large pastel of King David and Abishag, a young woman who was the old king's carer and concubine. Clotilde's image closely resembles the scene that is described over 200 pages earlier in the novel: 'Sur un fond de fleurs jetées, des fleurs en pluie d'étoiles, d'un luxe barbare, le vieux roi se présentait de face, la main posée sur l'épaule nue d'Abisaïg' ['Against a background of strewn flowers, a meteor shower of flowers, barbarous in its luxury, the old king stood face-on, his hand resting on Abisaïg's bare shoulder'].[67]

Clotilde's pastel is, as Harrow reminds us, 'an intentional pictorial translation of the fictional artist's relationship with her uncle; it figures the narrator's ekphrastic representation of the relationship between Pascal and Clotilde and it is the textual embodiment of the implied author's *reprise* of the original Biblical relation.'[68] If Harrow establishes the ekphrastic significance of Clotilde's Biblical pastel, then examining the novel from the perspective of the country doctor trope reveals the extent to which Pascal is seen as a local hero who assumes the positions of both God and sovereign. As Berger points out, given the isolation of the rural community which he serves, the country doctor is nothing less than a 'popular hero' who enjoys substantial local prestige.[69] Rothfield may lament that *Le*

[65] Zola, *Le Docteur Pascal*, p. 265.
[66] Ibid., p. 99.
[67] Ibid., p. 252.
[68] Harrow, *Zola, the Body Modern*, p. 102.
[69] Berger, *A Fortunate Man*, p. 165.

Médecin de campagne is a naïve utopian novel in which 'the physician rules as hero', but from the perspective of the doctor–patient relationship, the hero status of Benassis is crucial since it consolidates his position within the community.[70] Benassis is described by the villagers as possessing some God-like features: for example Jacquotte says that '[Benassis] fait quasiment des miracles dans l'endroit' ['[Benassis] practically performs miracles in the area'].[71] It is for this reason that Mireille Labouret persuasively argues for the prevalence of messianic imagery in the novel.[72] However, he is more often described as the people's hero. This hero-status certainly applies to Benassis, who is introduced as a *grand homme* from the beginning of the novel: 'cet homme est décidément un homme' ['this man is really a great man'][73] Benassis is also repeatedly compared to Napoleon, a significant honour since the village's only reference for contemporary affairs is Napoleon Bonaparte. But this comparison is given an important twist: just as Berger insists that the doctor is a *popular* hero, given his work with everyday people, Benassis is known as the 'Napoléon du peuple' ['Napoleon of the people'].[74]

The country doctor's relationship with his patients, based on an ethics of care and gratitude, thus serves as the basis from which the doctor establishes a relationship with the wider vicinity. This relationship with the local area is stronger in *Le Médecin de campagne* than in *Le Docteur Pascal*; nevertheless, both novels rely on the trope of the doctor's rounds to establish an image of the country doctor located within his community. These twinned features, the doctor's relationship with his patients and community, generate the myth of the doctor as a form of local hero. These two elements unite Benassis and Pascal even when their respective interests (reshaping the village and developing scientific theories) seem to divide them at first reading. That Benassis and Pascal are both at the intersection between these three elements suggests that they are both a 'fortunate man', as Berger's essay designates Sassall. However, in that essay Berger also points towards the anguish of the country doctor; his failures, his helplessness, and his own unhappiness that constantly threaten to overwhelm the country doctor.[75] To what extent do *Le Médecin de campagne* and *Le Docteur Pascal* also represent this darker side of the trope of the country doctor? By posing this question, I aim to tease out how the idealism and optimism surrounding the novels' portrayal of the country doctor are tinged with realism and pessimism. I argue that this combination of light and shade, of success and failure, of optimism

[70] Rothfield, *Vital Signs*, p. 47.
[71] Balzac, *Le Médecin de campagne*, p. 53.
[72] Mireille Labouret, 'De l'*Imitation de Jésus-Christ* à 'L'Évangile en action': images et paraboles dans *Le Médecin de campagne*', *L'Année balzacienne*, 4.1 (2003), 43–62.
[73] Balzac, *Le Médecin de campagne*, p. 25.
[74] Ibid., p. 213. 'Le Napoléon du peuple' is the title of chapter three of the novel.
[75] Berger, *A Fortunate Man*, p. 133.

and pessimism, is a central feature of the nineteenth-century literary country doctor.

Flaubert: Bovary, an Unfortunate *officier de santé*

Published twenty-three years after *Le Médecin de campagne*, and thirty-seven years before *Le Docteur Pascal*, Flaubert's *Madame Bovary* bridges Balzac's and Zola's novels and their respective depictions of country doctors and Flaubert's novel is an important step in the development of the doctor figure in the nineteenth-century realist imagination.[76] Although I will demonstrate that professional inadequacy and personal failure are integral to the trope of the country doctor in both *Le Médecin de campagne* and *Le Docteur Pascal*, equally significant is how these elements are framed by the novels' idealization of the doctor character, which will provide tragic contrast to the doctors' inevitable failures. In comparison, *Madame Bovary* focuses throughout on Bovary's personal and professional failures, with the exception of Rouault's broken leg which Bovary successfully sets. As Rothfield observes, *Le Médecin de campagne* contrasts to Flaubert's novel since the former depicts a utopic world dominated by a doctor-hero, whereas *Madame Bovary* represents 'a realistic world premised on the absence of [a] heroic physician.'[77]

Flaubert's novel suggests that his position as an *officier de santé* befits his (lack of) inner life. In Part One, Chapter Nine, the narration describes

> Charles, à la neige, à la pluie, chevauchait par les chemins de traverse. Il mangeait des omelettes sur la table des fermes, entrait son bras dans les lits humides, recevait au visage le jet tiède des saignées, écoutait des râles, examinait des cuvettes, retroussait bien du linge sale.[78]

> Charles, in the snow and rain, rode by side roads. He ate omelettes at farmhouse tables, put his arm into beds damp with sweat, had the lukewarm stream of bloodletting spurt into his face, listened to death rattles, examined the contents of bed pans, and hitched up a lot of filthy underclothes.

Using free indirect discourse to present Emma's view of Charles from the narrator's omniscient perspective, the passage relegates Charles's daily duties to nursing

[76] See Furst, 'Realism and Hypertrophy' for a reading of *Madame Bovary* alongside *Le Médecin de campagne* and *Le Docteur Pascal*. Flaubert was, famously, the son of a surgeon and there is an undeniable medical influence on both his work and how it has been received critically.

[77] Rothfield, *Vital Signs*, p. 47.

[78] Gustave Flaubert, *Madame Bovary: mœurs de province*, ed. by Thierry Laget (Paris: Gallimard, 2009), p. 114.

('retroussait bien du linge sale'), passive observation without decisive intervention ('écoutait des râles, examinait des cuvettes') as well as a proximity with the more repulsive aspects of medicine signalled by Charles's physical intimacy to feverish patients and their warm bodily fluids ('entrait son bras dans les lits *humides*, recevait au visage le jet *tiède* des saignées'; my emphasis). More significantly for our present focus, the doctor–patient relationship, central as it is to *Le Médecin de campagne* and *Le Docteur Pascal*, is abstracted in this passage since the patient is present only through objects relating to his or her illness, such as dirty laundry, blood, and bodily fluids. Instead, the passage focuses on the drudgery of Charles's life. Only the detail of him eating omelettes with his patients' families suggests a connection with the local community, but this is far from the gracious and earnest relationships seen in Balzac's and Zola's novels. Unlike Benassis and Pascal who, as will be evidenced, have an acute awareness of the limitations of their profession, Bovary exaggerates the importance of his duties: 'La nuit, quelquefois, Charles se réveillait en sursaut, croyant qu'on venait le chercher pour un malade: – J'y vais, balbutiait-il' ['Sometimes in the night, Charles would wake up with a start, believing that he was being looked for on behalf of a patient: "I'm coming," he would stammer'].[79]

Furthermore, although Bovary is a rural medical practitioner, he is neither a *médecin* or *docteur* as are Benassis and Pascal. Flaubert's novel makes much of Bovary's status as an *officier de santé*. Having failed his medical diploma, Bovary is resigned to assuming a lowlier medical position and his *Dictionnaire des sciences médicales* remains symbolically uncut.[80] In this way, *Madame Bovary* represents the historical introduction of the *officier de santé* position and the strict separation between the *officiers de santé* and their qualified medical counterparts, *médecins* and *docteurs*.[81] Bovary's humble position provides key sources of conflict in the novel: his lack of proper training is instrumental in his botching of Hippolyte's surgery, and his professional failures are thrown into sharper relief at the appearances of fully qualified medical doctors such as Doctor Canivet (a condescending surgeon from Neufchâtel who amputates Hippolyte's leg after the botched operation) and Doctor Larivière (a well-respected Rouennais doctor who attends Emma's bedside after she has swallowed arsenic). These differences between Flaubert on the one hand and Zola and Balzac on the other may be best explained by Flaubert's approach to medicine. As Rothfield observes, Flaubert was primarily interested in satirizing medicine in order appropriate its claim to objectivity for literary writing itself. The novel 'marks the emergence of a mode of writing in which the real has become medical, in which the relation between author and text is modelled on medical precepts, with the author viewing

[79] Flaubert, *Madame Bovary*, p. 189.
[80] Ibid., p. 81.
[81] Jacques Léonard, *La Vie quotidienne d'un médecin de province au XIXe siècle* (Paris: France Loisirs, 1993), pp. 68–80.

characters and situations as a doctor views patients and cases'.[82] At the same time that the novel is built on a logic that Rothfield construes as medical in nature, the novel explicitly denigrates medical science through what Furst terms as its 'reductive satire'.[83] Bovary's uncut dictionary thus 'thematises the determinate absence of medical knowledge. This knowledge—a system of presuppositions about illness and death—seems to be precisely what the novel excludes'.[84]

Flaubert's proclivity for medical satire is most evident in his representation of Doctor Larivière and his *regard médical* that supposedly dissects his patients: 'Son regard, plus tranchant que ses bistouris, vous descendait droit dans l'âme et désarticulait tout mensonge à travers les allégations et les pudeurs' ['His gaze, sharper than his scalpels, went straight through you and dissected every lie through allegation and modesty'].[85] Larivière is depicted as a tyrant whose dedicated students imitate his clothing (here we are reminded of the significance of the *robes noires* emphasized in *Le Médecin de campagne*) rather than his scientific prowess or bedside manner:

> Tout tremblait dans son hôpital quand il se mettait en colère, et ses élèves le vénéraient si bien, qu'ils s'efforçaient, à peine établis, de l'imiter le plus possible; de sorte que l'on retrouvait sur eux, par les villes d'alentour, sa longue douillette de mérinos et son large habit noir, dont les parements déboutonnés couvraient un peu ses mains charnues, de fort belles mains, et qui n'avaient jamais de gants, comme pour être plus promptes à plonger dans les misères.[86]

> Everything in his hospital shook when he got angry, and his students revered him so much that they tried to imitate him as much as possible, to such an extent that they were found, in the surrounding towns, wearing his long merino padded coat and his large black robe, of which the unbuttoned trim would barely cover his fleshy hands, his very beautiful hands, which never sported gloves, as if all the more ready to plunge into miseries.

Imitating the language of heroism, Larivière is described as 'Dédaigneux des croix, des titres et des académies, hospitalier, libéral, paternel avec les pauvres et pratiquant la vertu sans y croire' ['Disdainful of awards, titles, and academies; welcoming, liberal, fatherly with the poor and practising virtue without believing in it'].[87] Here the features integral to the country doctor trope, namely the doctor's

[82] Rothfield, *Vital Signs*, p. 37.
[83] Furst, 'Realism and Hypertrophy', p. 42.
[84] Rothfield, *Vital Signs*, p. 18. Interestingly, there is a notable lack of the medical characters in my corpus engaging with embedded texts, with the exception of Zola's Pascal who retreats into studying books rather than engaging with the practical side of his vocation.
[85] Flaubert, *Madame Bovary*, p. 413.
[86] Ibid., p. 413.
[87] Ibid., p. 413.

paternalism, philanthropism, and disdain for public recognition, are satirized by Flaubert's use of parataxis and the comment that the doctor practices virtue 'sans y croire' ['without believing in it']. *Madame Bovary* therefore appropriates the semantic fields heroism used to describe Benassis and Pascal: '[Larivière] eût presque passé pour un saint si la finesse de son esprit ne l'eût fait craindre comme un démon' ['Larivière] would almost have passed for a saint if the sharpness of his mind had not made him as feared as a devil'].[88] The deference that Larivière exacts is satirized through the other characters' reactions to him, even before he approaches the house: 'L'apparition d'un dieu n'eût pas causé plus d'émoi. Bovary leva les mains, Canivet s'arrêta court, et Homais retira son bonnet grec bien avant que le docteur fût entré' ['The appearance of a god would not have caused more excitement. Bovary raised his hands, Canivet stopped short, and Homais took off his Greek bonnet long before the doctor had entered'].[89] The use of the pluperfect subjunctive in these three instances ('eût passé', 'eût fait', 'fût entré') underlines the scene's satirical tone by drawing attention to what Larivière may have been similar, and the effect that he may have had had on the small group. Moreover, although Larivière is described with many of the hallmarks of the country doctor, the doctor–patient relationship is ironically displaced given Emma's near-death state by the time of the doctor's arrival. Her death a foregone conclusion, her relationship between Larrivière is superficial rather than therapeutic. Through its satire of the idealized country doctor trope, *Madame Bovary* lacks the idealist aesthetics associated with rural medicine, identified by Berger and plainly evident in Balzac and Zola. Nonetheless, Flaubert's novel points towards the inevitable failures that both Benassis and Pascal encounter during their professions and reminds us of the inherent limitations of the doctor–patient relationship when it is situated within the country doctor trope.

Balzac: Beneficence and Its Discontents

For all that it describes the country doctor as a quasi-mythical, idealized hero, Berger's essay also reveals this conception to be illusory. In reality, he writes, the fraternity between doctor and patient is not mutual, but rather it is 'an imaginative projection on Sassall's part', which thus makes him more a 'commander' of his patients than a brother.[90] This inherent asymmetry, Berger argues, leads to the country doctor's sense of personal and professional inadequacy, disillusionment with medicine, and a realization of the deep suffering that his patients experience.[91] The idealization of the country doctor is prone to inevitably give

88 Ibid., p. 413.
89 Ibid., p. 413.
90 Berger, *A Fortunate Man*, p. 111.
91 Ibid., pp. 112, 132, 165.

way to disenchantment and despair. Indeed, for all that *Le Médecin de campagne* portrays Benassis as a benevolent medical authority, the text thus throws light on the doctor's personal and professional failures, contributing to a more nuanced portrait of the country doctor. This section first analyses in more depth Benassis's claims about his role in reconstructing the village, and thus the ideas about authority that the text seemingly promulgates. I then examine key themes of the novel which undermine Benassis's claims about creating a medical utopia in the village, notably through his creation of the colony for sufferers of the congenital disease.

The figure of the failed hero is a familiar trope in *La Comédie humaine*, but Bernard Schilling claims that Benassis's turn to an apparent selfless project, rather than to suicide, sets him apart from the fate of more anguished protagonists such as Lucien de Rubempré.[92] Although Benassis's personal failures may not be as great as those of other Balzacian heroes, Carlos Testa persuasively argues for the failures within Benassis's utopic project that the text inadvertently reveals.[93] There are similar failures within the doctor–patient relationship: a breakdown of trust and a malfunctioning of the benevolent paternal authority on which the model of medicine detailed in the novel rests. Although Benassis decides not to take his own life, *Le Médecin de campagne* is far from a story of the country doctor's successful medical project.

The novel's third chapter focuses on a local dinner party with all the village's *robes noires* present: Benassis, the curé, the mayor, and the local justice of the peace. In nineteenth-century France, *robes noires* referred to members of the professional medical class who were characterized by the vocational aspect of their work. Middle-class professionals such as doctors, priests, and lawyers all wore black robes to signify their positions. Despite Benassis's earlier proclamation that the *robes noires* are united in their vocations to protect their local community, the dinner quickly descends into a heated discussion about the best way to administer the population. The discussion not only itself suggests the underlying tensions between the *robes noires*, pointing forwards to more serious fissures in the utopic village, but also allows Benassis to develop his ideas about his role in the local community through a series of extended monologues. Benassis opposes the idea of a middle-class revolution through democracy, fearing that it will eventually lead to a proletarian revolution. He says:

> Certes je crois avoir assez prouvé mon attachement à la classe pauvre et souffrante, je ne saurais être accusé de vouloir son malheur; mais tout en l'admirant dans la voie laborieuse où elle chemine, sublime de patience et de resignation, je

[92] Bernard N. Schilling, *The Hero as Failure: Balzac and the Rubempré Cycle* (Chicago, IL: University of Chicago Press, 1968), p. 61.

[93] Carlos Testa, 'The Sins of Utopia: Balzac's *Le Médecin de campagne*', *Nineteenth-Century French Studies*, 25 (1977), 280–92.

la declare incapable de participer au gouvernement. Les prolétaires me semblent les mineurs d'une nation, et doivent toujours rester en tutelle.[94]

Admittedly, I believe that I have sufficiently proved my attachment to the poor and suffering class; I cannot be accused of wanting this class's misfortune. But while admiring it in the labouring path that it walks, sublime in patience and resignation, I find this class incapable of participating in government. The proletariat seem to me to be the minors of a nation and must always remain in guardianship.

Here Benassis appeals to the intimacy with the poor that his profession lends him to justify a form of benevolent authoritarianism.[95] The evocation of 'mineurs' ['minors'] harks back to the deathbed scene with which *Le Médecin de campagne* opened, establishing that the maternalesque care with which Benassis treats his patients translates into quasi-paternal authoritarianism when it comes to administering the village. Indeed, the villagers refer to Benassis as 'notre père à tous' ['the father of everyone'], an epithet that is later engraved on his tombstone.[96] Chapter Two of this study tackles in more depth the question of the interconnectedness of paternal and medical authority.

Surprised at Benassis's ideas, Genestas presses the doctor to elaborate further. Benassis outlines a central social contract and a single authority to administer it. He justifies their superiority on the basis of what they give back to their community through their 'supériorité de pensée, supériorité politique, supériorité de fortune' ['superiority of thought, political superiority, and superiority of wealth'], and styles this arrangement as a form of social contract: 'Le contrat social, parlant de cette base, sera donc un pacte perpétuel entre ceux qui possèdent contre ceux qui ne possèdent pas. D'après ce principe, les lois seront faites par ceux auxquels elles profitent, cars ils doivent avoir l'instinct de leur conservation, et prévoir leurs dangers' ['The social contract, speaking of this basis, will therefore be a perpetual pact between the haves and the have-nots. According to this principle, the laws will be made by those whom they benefit because they must have the instinct of preserving themselves, and foresee any potential threats'].[97] Furthermore, this social contract should be, according to Benassis, administered by a central authority figure who benefits from a natural yet benevolent superiority over his community:

[94] Balzac, *Le Médecin de campagne*, p. 232.

[95] Benassis's appeal to his medical vocation to provide a mandate for civic authority, although Balzac's doctor scorns running for government, is echoed by Doctor Du Poirier in Stendhal's '*Lucien Leuwen*' during the doctor's speech made to Parliament: 'j'ai passé ces longues années à connaître les hommes de tous les rangs et à secourir le pauvre' ['I have passed these long years by getting to know men of all ranks and by helping the poor']. Stendhal, *Lucien Leuwen* (Paris: Gallimard, 2002), p. 657.

[96] Balzac, *Le Médecin de campagne*, p. 403.

[97] Ibid., p. 234.

> Le législateur [...] doit être supérieur à son siècle. Il constate la tendance des erreurs générales, et précise les points vers lesquels inclinent les idées d'une nation; il travaille donc encore plus pour l'avenir que pour le présent, plus pour la génération qui grandit que pour celle qui s'écoule. Or, si vous appelez la masse à faire la loi, la masse peut-elle supérieure à elle-même? Non.[98]

> The legislator [...] must be superior to his century. He notes the tendency of general errors, and specifies the points towards to which the ideas of a nation incline; so he works even more for the future than for the present; more for the future generation than for the present one. Now, if you call on the masses to create laws, can the masses be greater than themselves? No.

In these passages, the novel reimagines social relations by proposing a politics of care according to which the privileged are responsible for those who are less privileged, itself modelled on the doctor–patient relationship that provides the blueprint for the doctor's position within the community. Although these ideas are presented as belonging to Benassis, and his opinions are only gently contested by his fellow dinner party guests, the length and detail of his monologue give the impression that the system that the doctor proposes is one that the novel endorses. Yet, as Testa outlines, Benassis's views lead inevitably to totalitarianism under the guise of paternalism.[99] Elements of the novel thus undermine both the supposed social harmony of Benassis's system in addition to the idea that the doctor's monologue coincides with the agenda of the novel.

By referring to the social contract in addition to the figure of the Legislator, Balzac explicitly draws on Rousseau's ideas about social organization, and Anne-Marie Baron observes the importance of the idea of the social contract to both writers.[100] In *Le Contrat social*, Rousseau describes the Legislator as a superior being who constantly surveils his dependents: 'il faudrait une intelligence supérieure, qui vît toutes les passions des hommes et qui n'en éprouvât aucune' ['It would take a superior intelligence, which sees all the passions of men and yet feels none itself'].[101] The Legislator aims at transforming solitary humans into communal beings; altering subjects' constitutions with a view to strengthening them; and replacing the physical existence of nature with the moral existence of a higher plane.[102] His visionary sight supplements the blindness of those for whom he is responsible, aiding the 'multitude aveugle' ['blind masses'] by seeing on their behalf: 'De lui-même le peuple veut toujours le bien [...]. Il faut lui faire voir les

[98] Ibid., p. 235.
[99] Testa, 'The Sins of Utopia', p. 287.
[100] Anne-Marie Baron, 'Balzac et le *Contrat social* de Rousseau', *L'Année balzacienne*, 11.1 (2010), 249–65.
[101] Jean-Jacques Rousseau, *Du contrat social*, ed. by Bruno Bernardi (Paris: Flammarion, 2001), p. 79.
[102] Ibid., p. 80.

objets tels qu'ils sont' ['Of himself, the people always want the good [...]. We must make them see objects as they are'].[103] As such, the Legislator exercises reasoned judgement in order to create a just society: the Legislator 'est le mécanicien qui invente la machine' ['the mechanic that invents the machine'].[104] This idea of the creation of a utopic space is also echoed during Benassis's initial explanation of the village to Genestas, in which the doctor states that 'L'homme qui détruit et l'homme qui construit sont deux phénomènes de volonté' ['The man who destroys and the man who creates are two phenomena of will'].[105]

Beyond these direct references to Rousseauean discourse, *Le Médecin de campagne* also bears comparison with the system of beneficence, or *bienfaisance*, administered by Wolmar's estate at Clarens in *Julie, ou la Nouvelle Héloïse*. R. J. Howells comments that 'one can call Clarens a utopia in that it depicts a community living in optimum conditions, and because this is a closed society'.[106] For William Ray, the utopic depiction of Clarens extends to the level of the text itself: the novel 'does not merely represent the world, it proposes an ideal form of fictional discourse'.[107] Wolmar's Clarens estate is depicted as an ideal community, 'Tout y est agréable et riant, tout y respire l'abondance et la propreté, rien n'y sent la richesse et le luxe' ['Everything is pleasant and joyful, everything exudes abundance and cleanliness; nothing stinks of wealth or luxury'].[108] Wolmar pursues his aims through a system of beneficence which itself is praised in the novel as being at once good and beautiful: 'l'adorable et puissant empire que celui de la beauté bienfaisante!' ['the loveable and mighty empire of beneficent beauty!'].[109] Beneficence is best understood as a 'dynamic relationship which accepts *différence* and a real hierarchy' that works to 'minimise [social] hierarchy both by a kind of emotional fiction in the short term and by real change in the long term: the benefactor's supreme gift to the beneficiary is that the latter is enabled eventually to become a benefactor'.[110]

The idealized estate is construed in medical terms insofar as the economic and moral system of beneficence is used to metaphorically heal those within the system. Central to *La Nouvelle Héloïse* is the healing of Saint-Preux by his installation

[103] Ibid., p. 78.
[104] Ibid., p. 79.
[105] Balzac, *Le Médecin de campagne*, p. 90. Paulson persuasively argues that Balzac's utopic novel, through its oblique references to Rousseau's *Émile*, centres on Benassis's curing of Genestas's son, Adrien, of his mysterious illness, eventually identified as excessive masturbation. See Paulson, 'Preceptors, Fathers, and Ideology', p. 19.
[106] R. J. Howells, *Rousseau, Julie ou la Nouvelle Héloïse* (London; Wolfeboro, NH: Grant & Cutler, 1986), p. 39.
[107] William Ray, *Story and History: Narrative Authority and Social Identity in the Eighteenth-Century French and English Novel* (Oxford: Basil Blackwell, 1990), p. 241.
[108] Jean-Jacques Rousseau, *Julie, ou la Nouvelle Héloïse*, ed. by Henri Coulet, 2 vols (Paris: Gallimard, 1993), II, p. 55.
[109] Ibid., p. 58.
[110] Judith Still, *Justice and Difference in the Works of Rousseau*: Bienfaisance *and* Pudeur (Cambridge: Cambridge University Press, 1993), pp. 6–7.

on the estate and through his close contact with Wolmar, even though the latter is not a medical doctor. Echoing the doctor–patient relationship that is a founding site for the doctor's attempts to 'cure' his local community, the relationship that Wolmar creates between Saint-Preux, Julie, and all the estate's inhabitants cures their physical and moral ailments. Saint-Preux's installation at Clarens is therefore both his social and moral cure:

> Monsieur de Wolmar veut vous voir; il vous offre sa maison, son amitié, ses conseils: il n'en fallait pas tant pour calmer toutes mes craintes sur votre voyage, et je m'offenserais moi-même si je pouvais un moment me défier de vous. Il fait plus, il prétend vous guérir, et dit que ni Julie, ni lui, ni vous, ni moi, ne pouvons être parfaitement heureux sans cela.[111]

> Monsieur de Wolmar wants to see you; he offers you his home, his friendship, his advice: it didn't take so much to allay all my fears about your journey, and I would be offending myself if I didn't for a moment distrust you. He does more, he claims to heal you, and says that neither Julie, nor him, nor you, nor I, can be perfectly happy without that.

Wolmar is presented as a benevolent patriarch whose generous invitation into his home constitutes an essential physical and moral healing, indicated by the word *guérir* ['to heal']. Of note is also the emphasis on vision: Wolmar's insistence on the visual as a form of control also coincides with the conventional link made by contemporary materialist medical science between vision and understanding. In a similar vein, Andrea Goulet illustrates how the visual logic of Clarens embodies a Cartesian ideal of panoramic vision and transparent optics.[112] In this sense, Wolmar's visual power is the founding premise of his quasi-healing project.

Benassis's approach to healing the village works in a similar way to that of Wolmar's construction of Clarens. By recognizing the inequality between himself and his villagers, and indeed between the villagers, Benassis advocates for a model of benevolent paternalism that allows the privileged to take care of those who are less fortunate. Benassis hopes that those in positions of authority will inspire others, firstly, to live healthy and productive lives and, secondly, to become privileged caregivers themselves. Regarding the basketmaker he states: 'L'établissement de mon vannier était un exemple donné fructueusement à cette pauvre population' ['Establishing the basketmaker was a successful example for this poor population'].[113] The Rousseauian model of beneficence is thus given a medical twist in *Le Médecin de campagne*. Benassis aims to improve the health of the village through

[111] Rousseau, *Julie, ou, la Nouvelle Héloïse*, II, p. 28.
[112] Andrea Goulet, *Optiques: The Science of the Eye and the Birth of Modern French Fiction* (Philadelphia, PA: University of Pennsylvania Press, 2006), p. 69.
[113] Balzac, *Le Médecin de campagne*, p. 67.

economic and sexual productivity, embodied in the basketmaker's industriousness and marriage. The idea of healing the village finds its roots in the doctor–patient relationship, which serves as the model for Benassis's wider plans for the village. However, Benassis does not question or challenge the structures of social power relations, and instead uses the doctor–patient relationship to soften the worst aspects of them. In Chapters Two and Three, I will discuss in more detail how literary-medical encounters are used to challenge the asymmetric power structure of medicine as outlined by Benassis.

For all its idealized description, Wolmar's Clarens is not a perfect utopia: the success of Wolmar's system of beneficence is limited to the extent that is based on the principles of private property and subordination; its central limitation is its failure to be a genuine utopia built on the principles of beneficence.[114] There is also significant discontent within Benassis's village, despite his best attempts to cure it of its ills. These local grievances are first indicated after Benassis attends the bedside of the dying patient and are the originary point of Benassis's initial attempts to improve the village. Benassis explains that, when he first arrived in the village, he discovered a small colony of sufferers of the congenital disease alongside the able-bodied villagers, as well as the conditions that could cause 'cette contagion' ['this contagion'] to spread: 'La situation de ce hameau dans un fond sans courant d'air, près du torrent dont l'eau provient des neiges fondues, privé des bienfaits du soleil [...], tout y favorise la propagation de cette affreuse maladie' ['The situation of this hamlet in a valley without any wind, near the mountain stream whose water comes from the melted snow, deprived of the benefits of the sun [...]; everything here favours the spread of this cruel disease'].[115] This so-called unhealthy environment was fostered further by a local cult which believed that a colony would bring good luck to a neighbouring family.[116] Benassis then describes that he became mayor of the canton, paying a sizeable amount of money to transport them to Aiguebelle in the Savoie region in the dead of night.[117] The patient whose deathbed Benassis attends in chapter one is thus revealed to be the only one of his community who managed to escape the relocation and seek sanctuary within the village. John Mazaheri rightly points out that Benassis's forced relocation of the community, based on his prejudice against them, makes him an 'eugéniste *avant la lettre*' ['eugenicist *avant la lettre*'].[118] This episode thus throws new light on the scene of the patient's death with which *Le Médecin de campagne* opens, indicating that Benassis has not always been as generous to the patient and his community as the novel's deathbed scene suggests.

[114] See Still, *Justice and Difference in the Works of Rousseau*, pp. 75–7.
[115] Balzac, *Le Médecin de campagne*, pp. 41–2.
[116] Ibid., p. 42.
[117] Ibid., p. 42.
[118] John Mazaheri, *Essais sur la religiosité d'Honoré de Balzac* (Lewiston: Edwin Mellen Press, 2008), p. 35.

More than just revealing the village to be founded on a proto-eugenist principle, the episode also reveals significant discontent with Benassis's authority. Françoise Sylvos draws attention to similar fissures in the seemingly perfect utopia of the village.[119] Despite the doctor's intentions, the villagers are incensed at his attempts to cleanse the population and he laments that 'Aussitôt que cet acte d'humanité fut connu, je devins en horreur à toute la population' ['As soon as this act of humanity was known, I was loathed by the entire population'].[120] Here Benassis's use of the term 'humanité' contrasts sharply with his dehumanizing treatment of the group, revealing that the 'population' to which he refers, and accords value, is only the able-bodied villagers. Following the first forced relocation, Benassis's authority descends into tyranny. The local *curé* preaches against the doctor, so Benassis organizes for him to be replaced by the Bishop of Grenoble. The doctor's authoritarian control over the village as doctor-cum-mayor is also violently resisted by the villagers: a shot is fired by an unknown would-be assassin at the doctor in the local woods.[121] The doctors' proto-eugenicist crusade against the community, and the villager's strong reaction against it, throw new light on the trope of the country doctor. Rather than appearing as the monolithic 'popular hero' identified by Berger, Benassis's projects, despite his concern for the health of the village which eventually leads to the village's success, render him a highly contentious figure. By discriminating against the community, Benassis decides who does and does not qualify to enter the doctor–patient relationship with him. Foregrounding the extent to which the country doctor's medical practice may be discriminatory rather than universal, despite Benassis's appeal to the latter, suggests that the doctor is a gatekeeper of health rather than a neutral distributor of Rousseauean beneficence that seeks to heal equally every member of its community.

The representation of medicine is further complicated by what is later revealed of Benassis's own past. In chapter four, Benassis reveals his own life story and the reasons behind his dedication to the village. As Berger observes regarding Sassall and his anguish at his failure to help his patients, Benassis's story revolves around a similar emotion although it is caused by his personal rather than professional behaviour. Benassis says that, as a young man, he seduced a young woman who fell pregnant with his child. Both mother and child eventually died and, deeply repentant, Benassis entertained suicide before deciding that he needed to fulfil his desire to become an honourable 'chef de famille' ['head of the family'].[122] Benassis's confessions thus suggest that his relationship with patients, and indeed his entire project to heal the village, has been as much about healing

[119] Françoise Sylvos, 'La Poétique de l'utopie dans *Le Médecin de campagne*', *L'Annee balzacienne*, 4.1 (2003), 101–23.

[120] Balzac, *Le Médecin de campagne*, pp. 42–3.

[121] Ibid., p. 43.

[122] Ibid., p. 347.

himself. The doctor's attempt to heal his community through the doctor–patient relationship is thus a replacement for the failed father-son relationship he once enjoyed. *Le Médecin de campagne* thus suggests that the doctor–patient relationship is mutual, even if the doctor enjoys professional authority over the patient (which can be abused as in the case of Benassis). Finally, as mentioned in the Introduction of the present study, the *philosophe* Cabanis wrote that doctors should aim to ascend to a social and professional position similar to that of the priest: 'L'étude de l'homme physique est également intéressante pour le médecin et pour le moraliste: elle est presque également nécessaire à tous les deux' ['The study of the physical body is as interesting for the doctor as for the moralist: it is almost of equal importance for both'].[123] Benassis also aligns the role of medicine with that of the Church in his monologue on the *robes noires* mentioned above. The scene with Genestas, where the doctor confesses his errors, therefore undoes the role that Cabanis foresaw for doctors. Whereas Cabanis envisages the doctor assuming the role of the priest, in *Le Médecin de campagne* we see Benassis fashioning his interlocutor as a quasi-priest insofar as he asks Genestas to hear his confession.

On the one hand, *Le Médecin de campagne* frames Benassis's attempts to heal the *bourg* as founded in his personal life experience and a sense of paternal benevolence, in addition to an earnest attempt to heal himself. On the other hand, the violence inflicted on the colony, and thus the failure of Rousseauean beneficence, undermines this idealized portrait of the country doctor. Despite the novel's idealization of Benassis, at the same time it also suggests that the doctor acts, perhaps unwittingly, is the agent of an authoritarian normative regime (which, ironically, the doctor does not consider as his greatest sin). In short, then, the fact that Benassis's community is modelled on, and forged through, the doctor–patient relationship, means that the village is itself victim of the asymmetric power dynamic inherent to the medical relationship.

Zola: Professional Inadequacy and Doctor Pascal's *théorie dernière*

Berger characterizes the doctor's awareness of both medicine's failures and inevitable professional inadequacy as the quintessence of the country doctor. Berger argues that although all doctors experience helplessness when faced with failure, the country doctor is unique insofar as he chastises himself for mistakes which other doctors would classify as 'unfortunate complications', because of the patient's entire reliance on him as the only medical counsel they can receive.[124] The intimacy of the doctor–patient relationship also gives way to

[123] Cabanis, *Du degré de certitude*, p. vii.
[124] Berger, *A Fortunate Man*, p. 133.

what Berger frames as the suffering of the country doctor's patients and his failure to help them.[125] Comparable tendencies can be found in Zola's depiction of Doctor Pascal, taking us beyond both the quintessential understanding of him as a doctor-scientist as well as the novel's idealization of him as a country doctor.

Alongside the better-known *arbre généalogique*, Pascal is also interested in what the narrator styles as the dangerous *médecine des signatures*, discovered in a fifteenth-century medical textbook, which involves preparing a broth made from the organ of a sheep or cow corresponding to the organ responsible for a patient's illness, and then injecting that broth into the patient's arm.[126] The novel sees Pascal attending the deathbed of a local man, Lafouasse, after which Pascal returns home with a guilty conscience. The doctor is forebodingly described as 'bouleversé par un accident, ayant sur sa conscience de médecin aventureux la mort d'un homme' ['devastated by an accident, having on his conscience as a risk-taking doctor the death of a man'].[127] Pascal then recounts how Lafouasse's ataxia, a dysfunction of the nervous system, had left the patient all but doomed. Nonetheless, Pascal believes that his death was hastened and made more painful by his own clumsy intervention, recalling how he injected Lafouasse with an impure liquid, an accident revealed to him only when the patient immediately collapses from a suspected embolism. The narration describes how:

> le malheur avait voulu [...] que la petite seringue ramassât, au fond de la fiole, une parcelle impure échappée au filtre. Justement, un peu de sang avait paru, il venait, pour comble de malchance, de piquer dans une veine. Il s'était inquiété tout de suite, en voyant le cabaretier pâlir, suffoquer, suer à grosses gouttes froides. Puis, il avait compris, lorsque la mort s'était produite en coup de foudre, les lèvres bleues, le visage noir. C'était une embolie, il ne pouvait accuser que l'insuffisance de ses préparations, toute sa méthode encore barbare.[128]

> misfortune had wanted [...] the little syringe to pick up, at the bottom of the vial, an impure particle which had escaped the filter. At that moment, a little blood appeared; to make matters worse, he had just injected a vein. He was immediately worried, seeing the innkeeper turn pale, suffocate, break out in a cold sweat. Then he understood, when death suddenly struck: his blue lips, his darkened face. It was an embolism, and he could only blame the inadequacy of his preparations, his entire method that was still barbaric.

[125] Ibid., p. 112.
[126] Zola, *Le Docteur Pascal*, p. 92. Duffy argues that the injections are part of the incorporation of contemporary scientific discourse into the novel. See Duffy, *Flaubert, Zola*, pp. 194–217.
[127] Zola, *Le Docteur Pascal*, p. 189.
[128] Ibid., p. 190.

Lafouasse's painful death demonstrates that Pascal's ambitious medical experiments bear the risk of becoming iatrogenic, of the doctor inflicting illness or injury on his patient.[129] Written in free indirect discourse, blurring the boundary between narrative truth and character perception, the passage focuses less on the cause of Lafouasse's death, and more on the doctor's experience of professional inadequacy at the thought that he increased the suffering of a terminally ill patient. Pascal continues: 'Sans doute Lafouasse était perdu [...]; mais la brutalité du fait n'en était pas moins là, cette mort affreuse; et quel regret désespéré, quel ébranlement dans sa foi, quelle colère contre la science impuissante et assassine!' ['Without doubt Lafouasse was lost [...]; but the brutality of the fact was no less there—this dreadful death, and what desperate regret, what shock, what anger against powerless, murderous science!'].[130]

But Lafouasse's death is not the first time in *Les Rougon-Macquart* that Pascal has accidentally caused medical harm to one of his patients. As Schor observes, Pascal is haunted by the suicide of Albine in *La Faute de l'abbé Mouret*.[131] In that novel, Pascal allocates to Albine the caring responsibility for Serge Mouret, a young priest who suffers a nervous breakdown and amnesia induced by his religious fervour. Sequestered in the derelict estate of Le Paradou, Serge and Albine slowly fall in love and eventually consummate their relationship. The discovery of their relationship by Serge's former monsignor restores his memory to him and wracked with guilt at his carnal sins, Serge plunges more fervently into his faith. He then neglects Albine who eventually kills herself at the loss of Serge. Reflecting on this medical tragedy, Pascal acknowledges that he failed to adequately supervise her, favouring scientific study over his own caregiving duties: 'Il est vrai que [...] je n'ai pas bougé de mon laboratoire. J'avais des études en train... Et c'est ma faute!' ['It's true that [...] I have not left my laboratory. I had some studies in progress... And it's my fault!'].[132]

The medical harm eventually done to patients such as Lafouasse and Albine encourages a reconsideration of the opening chapter of *Le Docteur Pascal*. This chapter is well known for its image of the eponymous doctor sequestered in his study: 'Dans la chaleur de l'ardente après-midi de juillet, la salle, aux volets soigneusement clos, était pleine d'un grand calme. [...] Debout devant l'armoire, en face des fenêtres, le docteur Pascal cherchait une note' ['In the heat of an ardent afternoon in July, the room, with its carefully closed shutters, was filled with a great calm. [...] Standing in front of the cupboard, opposite the windows, Doctor Pascal was looking for a note'].[133] However, almost as soon as this image of

[129] For the term 'iatrogenesis', see Ivan Illich, *Limits to Medicine. Medical Nemesis: The Expropriation of Health* (London: Calder & Boyars, 1975), pp. 17–26.
[130] Zola, *Le Docteur Pascal*, p. 190.
[131] Schor, *Zola's Crowds*, p. 21.
[132] Zola, *La Faute de l'abbé Mouret*, p. 297.
[133] Zola, *Le Docteur Pascal*, p. 53.

Pascal is introduced is it disrupted by the doctor's medical failures. Pascal's mother Félicité, with whom he lives, violently accuses the doctor as responsible for the recent death of one of his patients, a local man named Boutin: 'Que fabrique-t-il donc, mon Dieu! Tu sais qu'il se fait le plus grand tort, avec sa drogue nouvelle. On m'a raconté que, l'autre jour, il avait encore failli tuer un de ses malades' ['What is he making, my God! You know he's doing the greatest harm to himself with his new drug. I was told the other day that he almost killed one of his patients again'].[134] On first reading, these accusations are presented as the hysterical ravings of the Zolian trope of the *dévote*, a woman unduly influenced by the Catholic Church, indicated by Félicité's appeal to God. But if we bear in mind the deaths of Albine and Lafouasse, both caused by Pascal's own failed interventions or neglect, Félicité's suspicions demand to be taken more seriously. Indeed, a few pages after Félicité's initial accusation, we find her accusation corroborated by Martine, the servant. Martine claims that that she believes that Félicité is right to be suspicious, and provides the reader with the crucial evidence. She says: 'Mme Félicité avait raison, hier, de dire qu'il y a vraiment de quoi rougir... On m'a jeté à la figure, à moi qui vous parle, qu'il avait tué le vieux Boutin, vous vous souvenez, ce pauvre vieux qui tombait du haut mal et qui est mort sur une route' ['Yesterday Mme Félicité was right to say that there really is something to be ashamed of... It was thrown in my face—me, who's talking to you now—that he killed old Boutin, you remember, this poor old man who fell from a great height and died on the road below'].[135] Boutin's sudden death is poorly explained by Pascal as being caused by a chronic condition, that he was 'un épileptique qui a succombé dans une crise congestive' ['an epileptic who succumbed to a congestive seizure'], but this reasoning seems ever more doubtful on second reading.[136]

If Pascal's failure to protect his patients from the potentially fatal consequences of his experimental medicine is a primary focus of *Le Docteur Pascal*, then the novel also sheds light on the country doctor's constant struggle to protect his patients from the violence that they inflict on themselves. A notable example from *A Fortunate Man* is that of suicide. Berger notes how, as a young doctor, Sassall was so preoccupied with the heroism of medicine that he could not recognize his patients' quotidian suffering amongst the more exciting emergencies. Berger thus outlines that 'A man who had never been ill shot his brains out' changed Sassall's approach to rural medicine.[137] The elliptical phrasing of this assertion, and its placement at the end of a paragraph by Berger, point towards the suicide's violence and inexplicability. *Le Docteur Pascal* contains a comparable event. The idyllic walk taken by Pascal and Clotilde in chapter eight is disrupted by the couple bumping into Sarteur, a milliner with a history of mental illness, who swears that

[134] Ibid., p. 64.
[135] Ibid., p. 85.
[136] Ibid., p. 95.
[137] Berger, *A Fortunate Man*, p. 55.

'il était tout à fait guéri de cette brusque rage homicide' ['he was completely cured of this sudden murderous rage'] by Pascal's treatment.[138] The doctor and Clotilde are both assured that Sarteur is healed, and his name only reappears in chapter twelve when Pascal is informed abruptly of his suicide. The sudden, tragic news forces Pascal to reconfront his professional inadequacy, and Pascal retraces how his previous belief, that his hypodermic injections had cured Sarteur of madness, was mistaken:

> Toute la soirée, il songea à ce cas étrange, à cet homme qu'il croyait avoir sauvé de la folie homicide, par sa médication des piqûres hypodermiques, et qui, évidemment, repris d'un accès, avait eu assez de lucidité encore pour s'étrangler, au lieu de sauter à la gorge d'un passant. Il le revoyait, si parfaitement raisonnable, pendant qu'il lui conseillait de reprendre sa vie de bon ouvrier. Quelle était donc cette force de destruction, le besoin du meurtre se changeant en suicide, la mort faisant sa besogne malgré tout? Avec cet homme disparaissait son dernier orgueil de médecin guérisseur; et, chaque matin, quand il se remettait au travail, il ne se croyait plus qu'un écolier qui épelle, qui cherche la vérité toujours, à mesure qu'elle recule et qu'elle s'élargit.[139]
>
> All evening he thought of this strange case, of this man whom he believed to have saved from homicidal madness by his medication of hypodermic injections, and who, evidently, having recovered from a fit, had still enough lucidity to strangle himself, instead of jumping at the throat of a passer-by. He saw him again now, seemingly perfectly calm, and he could see himself advising him to resume his life as a good work. What then was this destructive force, this need for murder that turned into suicide, death having its way despite everything? With this man disappeared his [Pascal's] last pride as a healer; and, every morning, when he got back to work, he thought of himself as a schoolboy who spells words out, who always searches for the truth that recedes and widens.

Sarteur's suicide suggests the extent to which Pascal's patients suffer physically from his failure to intervene in moments of mental and emotional crises. Pascal's question, 'Quelle était donc cette force de destruction?' ['So what was this destructive force?'], goes unanswered. Sarteur's suicide thus marks the lowest ebb of Pascal's professional self-esteem, rejecting his ideal of a *médecin guérisseur* which he replaces with a portrait of himself as an ignorant schoolboy. Berger's analysis of the country doctor suggests to us how Pascal's position, torn between a desire for absolute scientific knowledge and professional anguish at his responsibility for the harm caused by his experiments' failures, is the perpetual paradox of the country doctor.

[138] Zola, *Le Docteur Pascal*, p. 258.
[139] Ibid., p. 360.

After Lafouasse's death, Pascal withdraws entirely from his medical practice. Pascal's guilt leads him to reject even self-treatment when he falls ill, and he swears to never treat a patient again: 'Il niait la médecine, il jurait de ne plus toucher à un malade' ['He renounced medicine, he swore to not touch an ill person again'].[140] The failures of his scientific project, uncovered in the novel's first 300 pages, provoke clear disillusionment with his usual medical practice. Despite this dramatic rejection of medicine, and even the death of the eponymous hero a few pages from the novel's close, *Le Docteur Pascal* moves towards a triumphant ending that sees Pascal create and embrace a new vision of rural medicine, styled by the text as his 'théorie dernière' ['final theory']. Similarly to the utopianism of *Le Médecin de campagne*, Pascal's theory has not been well received by critics. Observing the utopian optimism in Zola's later works, F. W. J. Hemmings argues that 'with the exception of Sandoz in *L'Œuvre*, [Zola] never created a character more specifically charged with the function of expressing his own ideas. Sandoz gives us Zola's philosophy of art; Pascal his philosophy of life.'[141] Hemmings laments Zola's flight into scientific idealism: 'In *Le Docteur Pascal* all the tried principles by the application of which Zola had achieved integrated and lofty works of art are rejected: objectivity, irony, the adherence to logical determinism, the refusal to philosophise and to read a sermon into the study of human nature.'[142] The novel marks a departure from the realist tone of *Les Rougon-Macquart* and heralds the beginning of Zola's idealistic period: *Le Docteur Pascal* was published while Zola conceived and began work on his *romans à thèse*. Rather than seeing *Le Docteur Pascal* as less sober than Zola's previous novels, here I reread Pascal's theory of the asymmetric doctor–patient relationship, which finds echoes in both *Le Médecin de campagne* and the Rousseauean ideas of beneficence, in order to argue that a form of inequality that is both benevolent and paternal is at the heart of the relationship between country doctor and patient. By taking seriously the final chapters of *Le Docteur Pascal*, I build on David Baguley's attempts to reconcile Zola's recourse to utopianism with his earlier Naturalist mode.[143]

As mentioned previously, Pascal grows increasingly dissatisfied with the scientific view of medicine that once led him to experiment with hypodermic injections. Whereas he previously considered his medical rounds 'des tournées de miracles' ['miracle rounds'],[144] he now confesses to Clotilde that he only finds them 'des tournées de soulagement et de consolation' ['alleviation and consolation

[140] Ibid., p. 204.
[141] F. W. J. Hemmings, *Émile Zola* (Oxford: Clarendon Press, 1966), p. 257.
[142] Ibid., p. 258.
[143] David Baguley, 'Du récit polémique au discours utopique: l'Évangile républicain de Zola', *Cahiers naturalistes*, 54 (1980), 106–21. The contrast between Zola's early and late work leads Henri Mitterand to speak of a fourth Zola. See Henri Mitterand, 'Le Quatrième Zola', *Œuvres et critiques*, 16.2 (1991), 85–98.
[144] Zola, *Le Docteur Pascal*, p. 98.

rounds']. [145] Pascal delves into his medical library in the hope of excitedly throwing himself back into medical practice once he isconfident of the success of his hypodermic injections, only to be once again disappointed. Pascal is now aggrieved by empiricism and feels the emptiness of medical therapeutics: 'il sentait tout le vide de la thérapeutique. L'empirisme le désolait' ['he felt all the emptiness of therapeutics. He was saddened by empiricism']. [146] Although Pascal still believes in the importance of driving medicine towards an experimental method, he laments the numerous patients' deaths caused by their doctors' futile searches for new cures:

> Du moment que la médecine n'était pas une science expérimentale, mais un art, il demeurait inquiet devant l'infinie complication de la maladie et du remède, selon le malade. Les médications changeaient avec les hypothèses: que de gens avaient dû tuer jadis les méthodes aujourd'hui abandonnées! [147]
>
> As long as medicine was not an experimental science but an art, he was worried about the endless complications of disease and cure, depending on the patient. Treatment changed according to assumptions: how many people, in the past, had had to kill off the methods that had already been abandoned today!

Pascal begins to understand that, from the patient's perspective, the only certain element of the medical encounter is the doctor's presence. As such, 'Le flair du médecin devenait tout, le guérisseur n'était plus qu'un devin heureusement doué, marchant lui-même à tâtons' ['The doctor's flair became everything, the healer was nothing more than a happily gifted diviner, groping his way in the dark']. [148] Notwithstanding this assertion's appeal to notions of medical genius, what is most important according to Pascal is that the doctor is perceived as a genius by the patient. This perception has the effect that being injected with water is equally as effective as being injected with Pascal's special *liqueur*. Having realized as much, and now disillusioned with experimental medicine, Pascal abandons all his patients except those 'qui le réclamaient à grand cris et qui se trouvaient miraculeusement soulagés, même lorsqu'il les piquait avec de l'eau claire' ['who cried out for him and found themselves miraculously relieved, even when he injected them with clean water']. [149]

Le Docteur Pascal here echoes contemporary opinion on the importance of the placebo effect to cure patients. Jules Chéron acknowledged in his *Introduction à l'étude des lois générales de l'hypodermie, physiologie et thérapeutique* that 'Toutes

[145] Ibid., p. 264.
[146] Ibid., p. 264.
[147] Ibid., p. 264.
[148] Ibid., pp. 264–5.
[149] Ibid., p. 265.

les injections hypodermiques produisent des effets identiques quelle que soit le liquide introduit sous la peau, à la condition que ce liquide ne soit pas toxique. La différence ne porte que sur l'intensité plus ou moins grande du phénomène produit' ['All hypodermic injections produce identical effects regardless of the liquid introduced under the skin, provided that this liquid is not toxic. The difference only relates to the greater or lesser intensity of the phenomenon produced'].[150] Rather than 'Guérir, retarder la mort' ['Cure, delay death'] as his old mantra proclaimed, Pascal now concludes that healing is tantamount to the relieving of suffering: 'Ah! soulager, empêcher la souffrance, cela, certes, je le veux encore! [...] Je ne soigne plus que pour empêcher la souffrance' ['Ah, relieving, preventing suffering, that I still want of course! [...] I only heal to prevent suffering'].[151]

The importance placed on healing (*soulager*) over curing (*guérir*) eventually leads to Pascal's 'théorie dernière', espoused some hundred pages later.[152] In a quasi-confessional scene, Pascal theorizes to a colleague, Doctor Ramond, that 'L'homme baignait dans un milieu, la nature, qui irritait perpétuellement par des contacts les terminaisons sensitives des nerfs' ['Man was immersed in an environment, nature, which perpetually irritated the sensitive nerve endings by contact with them'], producing internal and external sensory experiences, concluding that health depends on the correct balance of sensations.[153] For Pascal, medical treatment therefore constitutes the re-establishment of an equilibrium within the body reminiscent of vitalist, materialist, and deist equilibrium approaches: 'il avait la conviction que se bien porter consistait dans le train normal de ce travail: recevoir les sensations, les rendre en idées et en mouvements, nourrir la machine humaine par le jeu régulier des organes' ['he was convinced that being in good health was a normal part of his job: receiving sensations, rendering them into ideas and movements, nourishing the human machine through the regular rhythm of the organs'].[154] Pascal's final theory builds on the original design of the hypodermic injections, which depend on the principle of the circulation of blood. Much earlier in the novel the narrator notes that

> [Pascal] croyait avoir découvert la panacée universelle, la liqueur de vie destinée à combattre la débilité humaine, seule cause réelle de tous les maux, une véritable et scientifique fontaine de Jouvence, qui, en donnant de la force, de la santé et de la volonté, referait une humanité toute neuve et supérieure.[155]

[150] Jules Chéron, *Introduction à l'étude des lois générales de l'hypodermie, physiologie et thérapeutique* (Paris: Société d'éditions scientifiques, 1893), pp. 61–62.

[151] Zola, *Le Docteur Pascal*, pp. 260, 261. Carol A. Mossman observes that Zola elsewhere valorizes the pain of childbirth, in *Politics and Narratives of Birth: Gynocolonization from Rousseau to Zola* (Cambridge; New York: Cambridge University Press, 1993), pp. 208–16.

[152] This preference for healing over curing echoes the assertion made by Bianchon in *Le Père Goriot*: 'nous ne guérissons pas, nous aidons à guérir' ['we do not heal, we facilitate healing']. See Balzac, *Le Père Goriot*, p. 292.

[153] Zola, *Le Docteur Pascal*, p. 376.

[154] Ibid., p. 376.

[155] Ibid., p. 97.

> [Pascal] believed that he had discovered the universal panacea, the liquor of life intended to combat human debility, the only real cause of all ills, a real and scientific elixir of youth which, by giving strength, health, and will, would make a new and superior humanity.

Following the trauma of his patients' deaths, Pascal now contends that life consists of man's immersion in his environment, which animates 'la machine humaine' ['the human machine'], concluding that 'Le travail devenait ainsi la grande loi, le régulateur de l'univers vivant' ['Work thus became the great law, the regulator of the living universe'].[156] In Chapter Four I return to Zola's interest in eighteenth-century conceptions of vital fluids.

Although this assertion echoes Zola's interest in the experimental method insofar as both posit that the writer-doctor must study how environment shapes its subjects, Pascal also pays attention to the interpersonal side of his new medical theory. He theorizes that illness is caused by changes in the environment that disrupt the body's natural balances, and thus formulates an entirely new system for healing:

> [Pascal] rêvait toute une médication nouvelle: la suggestion, *l'autorité toute-puissante du médecin* pour les sens; l'électricité, les frictions, le massage pour la peau et les tendons; les régimes alimentaires pour l'estomac; les cures d'air, sur les hauts plateaux, pour les poumons; enfin, les transfusions, les piqûres d'eau distillée pour l'appareil circulatoire. *C'était l'action indéniable et purement mécanique* de ces dernières qui l'avait mis sur la voie, il ne faisait qu'étendre à présent l'hypothèse, par un besoin de son esprit généralisateur, il voyait de nouveau le monde sauvé dans cet équilibre parfait, autant de travail rendu que de sensation reçue, le branle du monde rétabli dans *son labeur éternel.*
>
> (My emphasis.)[157]

> [Pascal] dreamed of a new form of medication: suggestion, *the doctor's omnipotent authority* for the senses; electricity, friction, and massage for the skin and tendons; diets for the stomach; taking mountain air for the lungs; finally, transfusions, injections of distilled water for the circulatory system. *It was the undeniable and purely mechanical action* of the latter that had set him on the path, he was only now extending the hypothesis; by a need of his generalizing mind, he saw again the world saved in this perfect balance, as much work returned as sensation received, the movement of the world re-established in *its eternal labour.*
>
> (My emphasis.)

[156] Ibid., p. 376.
[157] Ibid., pp. 376–7.

Here, the 'flair du médecin', originally formulated 100 pages previously, is converted into the all-powerful authority of the doctor who heals his patient through suggestion: the other cures purport to the doctor's ability to manipulate the exterior and interior of the patient's body. The pervading semantic field of mechanism and labour, linked to the human 'mécanisme' evoked in 'Le Roman expérimental' ('action', 'mécanique', 'labeur'); as well as a lexicon of religious authority ('autorité toute-puissante', 'indéniable', 'purement', 'éternel') combine to produce an image of an all-knowing, all-healing, vitalist country doctor. Despite the doctor's authority within this scheme, the patient is at the implicit centre of this passage: the complex medical interventions described are all in relation to the diseased body. Thus, in Pascal's new medicine, the success of the patient's healing experience would be defined by the extent to which the placebo injection soothes their pain, since it is the combination of medication and its administration that heals.

The foregrounding of the healing potential of the doctor's presence coincides with concepts in the medical humanities, such as Balint's concept of the 'atmosphere' that surrounds the doctor and that he controls:

> By far the most frequently used drug in general practice was the doctor himself. It was not only the bottle of medicine or the box of bills that mattered, but the way that the doctor gave them to his patient—in fact, the whole *atmosphere* in which the drug was given and taken
>
> (Emphasis original.)[158]

The new medicine formulated in *Le Docteur Pascal* thus relies on a model of an asymmetric power dynamic between country doctor and patient, and that this relationship is governed by a principle of paternal benevolence. Like Zola in *Le Docteur Pascal*, Berger also acknowledges that, firstly, the patient is the 'central character' of the doctor–patient relationship, and secondly, that the medical outcome depends on the doctor's 'sense of mastery' of the otherwise fraught medical encounter.[159] This mastery is derived from the doctor's thirst for knowledge, reminiscent of Pascal's own study: Sassall's self-identification as a 'Master Mariner' is driven by his curiosity towards the patient's body.[160] Despite the doctor's best intentions to create an atmosphere of mutuality around the doctor–patient relationship, Sassall is aware that his mastery is built on a fundamental inequality between doctor and patient that fraternal sentiment cannot overcome. Berger thus identifies that the inequality between patient and country doctor, between the patient's acceptance of their lot in life and the doctor's constant striving to learn more, is the central, but unequal dynamic, on which the medical relationship depends:

[158] Balint, *The Doctor, His Patient, and the Illness*, p. 1.
[159] Berger, *A Fortunate Man*, p. 77.
[160] Ibid., p. 80.

> [The patient's] backwardness enables him to follow his cases through all their stages, grants him the power of his hegemony, encourages him to become the 'consciousness' of the district, allows him unusually promising conditions for achieving a 'fraternal' relationship with his patients, permits him to establish almost entirely on his own terms the local image of his profession. [...] Sassall can strive towards the universal because his patients are underprivileged.[161]

By accepting the inherent asymmetry of the doctor–patient relationship, Pascal responds to his patients' need for emotional support in a way that redeems both them and himself through a form of measured medical paternalism. Pascal's *théorie dernière* is thus tantamount to an acceptance, or even the promotion, of the doctor's authority over that of the patient. However, the origin of the doctor's authority is perhaps unexpected: in *Le Docteur Pascal*, the eponymous doctor's position of privilege over the patient comes from his knowledge not of scientific medicine, as the opening chapters of the novel initially suggest, but of the pain and suffering inherent to life itself. For Zola, as for Berger, then, the country doctor understands and recognizes his patient through mutual suffering, and it is this understanding that serves as the basis for what the novel presents as the necessarily asymmetric doctor–patient relationship. Despite the critical commonplace that *Le Docteur Pascal* represents the apogee of Zola's quasi-scientific novel, the eponymous doctor can also be read as being part of a long line of literary country doctors who display characteristics such as self-doubt and anguish. Despite Zola's and Balzac's insight into the challenges that the country doctor may face, these obstacles only serve to further cement the doctor's paternal ascendancy over the patient.

Conclusion

In *Le Médecin de campagne* and *Le Docteur Pascal*, the nineteenth-century country doctor is characterized by, firstly, his connection to the patient, articulated through the specificity and depth of the doctor–patient relationship; secondly, his connection to the locale, indicated by scenes that serve to root the doctor in either his community or landscape. These two features combine to produce the third and most striking category of the country doctor: the characterization of the country doctor as an ideal popular hero. Both *Le Médecin de campagne* and *Le Docteur Pascal* rely on religious imagery and semantics to idealize the doctor, sharply contrasting with the secular image of medicine that a modern-day reader may expect. Idealism is essential to the trope of the country doctor: without idealism, a desire to make the world a better place, the anguish of the country

[161] Ibid., p. 144.

doctor is less sorely felt. In *Le Médecin de campagne*, the hierarchy of the doctor–patient relationship is both medicine's strength and its downfall. The irony at play, namely the fact that the doctor–patient relationship is both at the centre of Benassis's project and undermines it, reveals Balzac's ambivalence towards the practice of medicine. By contrast, *Le Docteur Pascal* turns towards a reaffirmation of the doctor–patient relationship, recharacterizing Pascal as a practising doctor rather than a scientist. The doctor–patient relationship is thus at the centre of the literary trope of the country doctor, foregrounding the interpersonal dynamic of medicine over its scientific dimension. The medical relationship is frequently elided with the encounter, since the latter is presented as a symptom of the former that allows us to understand the special nature of the relationship between the country doctor and his patients. Furthermore, the nineteenth-century French trope of the country doctor throws new light on the doctor–patient relationship itself. Whereas the medical relationship is most often understood as an interpersonal relationship between two people, this chapter illustrates that it can also operate as a blueprint for a more abstract relationship between the doctor and his local community.

The literary trope of the country doctor seen here is profoundly conservative: by pointing out the doctor's flaws, both *Le Médecin de campagne* and *Le Docteur Pascal* justify a paternalistic model of medicine that styles the doctor as the ultimate authority over the patient. The dominance of the doctor relies on ableist discourse: by characterizing the sufferers of a congenital disease as less than human, the novel paradoxically portrays Benassis as both sympathetic to them (in the opening doctor–patient encounter) but also as embarking on a proto-eugenist policy against them. The following two chapters on Stendhal's *Lamiel* and Sand's *Lélia* respectively both articulate how the (often female) patient questions, undermines, and resists this form of medical paternalism. What this chapter has attempted to establish is that novels are as invested in the doctor's so-called natural authority as they are his scientific authority. In the two subsequent chapters, we shall see that both forms of authority are called into question.

Chapter Two
Blood at the Bedside: Subverting the Medical Relationship in Stendhal

Introduction

In Chapter One we saw how Balzac's and Zola's novels depict medical relationships that generally adhere to the conventional binarism and hierarchy power dynamic between both doctor and patient. This benevolent form of medical paternalism is idealized as a way that doctors can save their patients, their local communities, and thus themselves. Moreover, we saw how the bedside encounter was often taken to be a metonymy for the doctor–patient relationship itself. Despite the idealism of these representations of rural medical practice, this form of medical paternalism is not uncontested: as Elsner persuasively argues, novels consistently undermine this form of authority thanks to their textual slipperiness and their entanglement with a myriad of antagonistic discourses and perspectives.[1] In this chapter, I illustrate how these elements of the doctor–patient relationship are challenged and undermined by medical encounters in two of Stendhal's novels, *Lamiel* and *Lucien Leuwen*.

Unlike Balzac and Zola, Stendhal is not often considered to be a medically or scientifically minded writer: Jean Théodoridès describes the scientific aspect of Stendhal's work as 'peu connu et jusqu'ici non étudié' ['poorly known and unstudied up until now'], even though 'Chez Stendhal, cet intérêt pour les questions scientifiques est encore plus vif [que chez Balzac ou chez Flaubert]' ['With Stendhal, this interest in scientific questions was more lively [than with Balzac or Flaubert]'].[2] His major novels, *Le Rouge et le Noir* and *La Chartreuse de Parme* feature no central medical characters. Instead, these texts make religious and paternal authority the main figures of their critique. Although both *Lucien Leuwen* and *Lamiel* feature important doctors, these novels have both received significantly less scholarly attention given their statuses as unfinished works and thence their relative marginal position in Stendhal's œuvre.[3] My primary object of study in this chapter is the final substantial version of *Lamiel*, written in 1840; the final section of this chapter compares *Lamiel* to *Lucien Leuwen*.

[1] Anna Magdalena Elsner, 'Beyond Medical Paternalism: Undoing the Doctor-Patient Relationship in Simone de Beauvoir's A Very Easy Death', *Literature and Medicine*, 37.2 (2019), p. 422.

[2] Jean Théodoridès, *Stendhal du côté de la science* (Aran: Éditions du Grand chêne, 1972), p. 10.

[3] See ibid., pp. 209–12 and pp. 219–23 for a summary of the encounters with doctors and illnesses in *Le Rouge et le Noir* and *La Chartreuse de Parme* respectively.

The Doctor–Patient Relationship and the Nineteenth-Century French Novel. Sarah Jones, Oxford University Press.
 DOI: 10.1093/oso/9780198893790.003.0003

Lamiel depicts the eponymous heroine, a young Norman peasant girl, after she is sent to the local castle to work as a *lectrice* for the *châtelaine*. She encounters Doctor Sansfin after falling ill with an ambiguous mix of both ennui and tuberculosis: a cocktail of illness that I will explore in more detail. On the one hand, some critics characterize Sansfin as a domineering doctor, especially when focusing on the latest significant manuscript, they have often characterized *Lamiel* as a novel of masculine domination through medical malpractice. For example, Dennis Porter argues that in this scene Lamiel is 'disturbed in such a way as to suggest an apprehension inspired by what is, in effect, a parodic but cruel enactment of sexual relations with Sansfin'.[4] According to this reading, the doctor–patient relationship between Sansfin and Lamiel is thus asymmetric and hierarchical: Lamiel is slowly effaced from the novel as she is overwhelmed by Sansfin. On the other hand, critics such as Naomi Schor, Lucy Garnier, and Maria Scott foreground Lamiel's uncontrolled sense of freedom in the earlier version of the novel, particularly her insatiable thirst for liberty.[5] These feminist interpretations of *Lamiel* focus on the manuscript's earlier substantial version, written between October and December 1839, rather than the second substantial version of the manuscript, composed in January 1840.[6] The Lamiel of the later manuscript version is generally understood to be a more 'limited creation' than her earlier incarnation.[7]

This chapter reconciles this feminist approach with the critical commonplace that the protagonist from the later manuscript is less daring than her earlier incarnations. It argues that the scene in which Lamiel pretends to cough up blood reveals an intricate doctor–patient relationship that sheds light on the role of Lamiel in the novel. Although Yves Ansel has argued that 'Isoler et privilégier la relation entre Lamiel et Sansfin, c'est *ipso facto* tronquer la lettre du texte' ['Isolating and privileging the relationship between Lamiel and Sansfin is *ipso facto* truncating the letter of the text'], this chapter argues that exploring the dynamic between doctor and patient in *Lamiel* reveals new ways to understand the medical, iconographic, and metaphorical texture of the novel.[8] I explore how *Lamiel* overturns the hierarchical and asymmetric doctor–patient relationship dominated by the paternal malevolence of the medical professional. This paternal medical relationship is undermined by an extraordinary encounter between doctor and patient, in which the latter manipulates a ruse proposed by the former in order to exact her own freedom. Although Sansfin may exhibit some characteristics of

[4] Dennis Porter, '*Lamiel*: The Wild Child and the Ugly Men', *Novel: A Forum on Fiction*, 12.1 (1978), 21–32 (p. 26).

[5] Naomi Schor, *Breaking the Chain: Women, Theory, and French Realist Fiction, Gender and Culture* (New York: Columbia University Press, 1985); Maria Scott, *Stendhal's Less-Loved Heroines: Fiction, Freedom, and the Female* (London: Legenda, 2013); Lucy Garnier, 'La Femme comme construction dans la fiction stendhalienne' (DPhil thesis, University of Oxford, 2007), p. 131.

[6] For a full overview of the different critical responses to the two versions of *Lamiel* and the status of its manuscript, see Garnier, 'La Femme comme construction dans la fiction stendhalienne', pp. 114–20.

[7] Scott, *Stendhal's Less-Loved Heroines*, p. 85.

[8] Yves Ansel, *Stendhal littéral: 'Lamiel'* (Grenoble: ELLUG, 2009), p. 122.

a paternal and controlling doctor, I argue that Lamiel finds a way to rebel. In this chapter's final section I compare *Lamiel* to *Lucien Leuwen*, finding that although the novel presents a less radical subversion of the doctor–patient relationship, it nonetheless questions its binary nature.

Lamiel, Consumptive Heroine

Lamiel is rarely read as a novel concerned with illness and medicine: scholars who mention Lamiel's physical illness foreground either Sansfin himself, or the more ambiguous emotional distress from which Lamiel suffers. Discussing Lamiel's illness, Théodoridès foregrounds Sansfin's plot to influence the Duchesse and thus prioritizes the doctor's narrative thread over his patient's, implying the dominance of the former over the latter.[9] For his part, C. W. Thompson highlights only the mental health aspect of her illness: 'Anorexie, dégoût, spleen' ['Anorexia, repugnance, spleen'].[10] This failure to classify Lamiel as consumptive may partly be due to the Romantic trope of the wasting away of female sufferers of tuberculosis: Nancy Rogers asserts that French literature from the Romantic period is populated by the incremental, wasting deaths of 'the positive, sweet, worthy female figure who forms one side of the Romantic conception of womanhood', citing examples such as Rousseau's Julie, Stendhal's Madame de Rênal, and Sand's Valentine.[11] Despite her departure from this mode of tuberculous femininity, I argue here that Lamiel should be read as a consumptive patient and, in the following section, discuss how the novel subverts the trope of feminine wasting away in order to establish a new mode of female patienthood. Furthermore, recuperating Lamiel as a patient indicates the potential value of broadening our understanding of the doctor–patient relationship.

Despite this relative lack of scholarly interest in the illness of the eponymous heroine, Lamiel's consumptive state is stated clearly in both the novel and in Stendhal's notes. At fifteen years old, Lamiel is sent away by her adoptive aunt and uncle to work as a *lectrice* for the Duchesse de Miossens. As soon as she enters the castle that is to be her home and workplace, she falls seriously ill and begins exhibiting the hallmark symptoms of tuberculosis such as extreme paleness, ruddy cheeks, and, later, dramatic weight loss.[12] Deeply concerned by her poor health, the Duchesse calls for Sansfin to assess the patient. His diagnosis confirms that

[9] Théodoridès, *Stendhal du côté de la science*, pp. 227–8.

[10] C. W. Thompson, *Lamiel, fille du feu: essai sur Stendhal et l'énergie* (Paris: L'Harmattan, 1997), p. 23.

[11] Nancy Rogers, 'The Wasting Away of Romantic Heroines', *Nineteenth-Century French Studies*, 11.3/4 (1983), 246–56 (p. 252).

[12] Stendhal, *Lamiel*, in *Œuvres romanesques complètes*, ed. by Yves Ansel, Philippe Berthier, and Xavier Bourdenet, 3 vols (Paris: Gallimard, 2005–14), III (2014), ed. by Yves Ansel, Philippe Berthier, Xavier Bourdenet, and Serge Linkès, pp. 835–1094 (pp. 1003, 1005, 1082, 1083). Throughout this monograph I refer to the three-volume series of Stendhal's novelistic work as *ORC*.

Lamiel's symptoms are caused by consumption, alluding to 'l'effroyable maladie de poitrine' ['the terrible lung disease'].[13] Stendhal's preparatory notes for this version of the novel also suggest that Lamiel suffers from consumption: he writes that, once installed at the castle, Lamiel 'tomba malade' ['fell ill']; that she is 'malade de poitrine' ['ill in the chest']; and that she 'passait pour avoir un commencement de maladie de poitrine' ['seemed to be at the beginning of a chest condition'].[14] Stendhal even sketches out a scene wherein Sansfin 'vit la petite Lamiel venant à pied du château, elle qui, malade de poitrine et la favorite de Madame, ne marchait jamais qu'en voiture' ['saw the little Lamiel leaving the castle on foot, she who, suffering from chest condition and the favourite of Madame, only ever travelled by carriage'].[15]

The most important advance in the understanding of consumption during the early nineteenth century was that by René Laënnec, whose research on consumption had both an immediate and enduring effect on the medical community.[16] His treatise, *De l'auscultation médiate, ou traité du diagnostic des maladies des poumons et du cœur* was printed seven times in French between 1819 and 1839. Furthermore, it was widely cited by contemporary doctors are the most important text on tuberculosis until well into the 1860s, and the treatise was reprinted as late as 1879.[17] Although Laënnec's most important medical contribution was his revolutionization of the medical understanding of tuberculosis's physiology, through his novel unitary theory of the disease, his cultural legacy departs from his professional reputation as a close observer of the human body. Outside the medical world, Laënnec's legacy lies in his emphasis on how illness 'arose spontaneously from internal causes'.[18] According to Laënnec, the most important external cause of consumption was the presence of *passions tristes*: 'Parmi les causes occasionnelles de la phthisie pulmonaire, je n'en connais pas de plus certaines que les passions tristes, surtout quand elles sont profondes de longue durée' ['Among the occasional causes of phthisis of the lungs, I know none more certain than sad passions,

[13] Stendhal, *Œuvres romanesques complètes III*, ed. by Yves Ansel, Philippe Berthier, Xavier Bourdenet, and Serge Linkès, Bibliothèque de la Plèiade, 3 vols (Paris: Gallimard, 2014), III, p. 1004. Sansfin's elliptical allusion to consumption mirrors how the mother of Octave de Malivert in *Armance* refuses to 'nommer cette maladie cruelle', *ORC*, I, p. 91.

[14] Ibid., III, pp. 1076, 1082, 1088.

[15] Ibid., III, p. 1082.

[16] Jacalyn Duffin, *To See with a Better Eye: A Life of R. T. H. Laennec* (Princeton, NJ; Chichester: Princeton University Press, 1998), p. 211.

[17] In her biography of Laënnec, Duffin argues that his work had both an immediate and enduring effect on the medical community. Ibid., p. 211.

[18] David S. Barnes, *The Making of a Social Disease: Tuberculosis in Nineteenth-Century France* (Berkeley; London: University of California Press, 1995), p. 27. Here Barnes builds on the work of historians interested in his cultural legacy tend to characterize him as a 'Romantic' or 'essentialist' writer. However, for the problematic use of the term 'Romantic' medicine, which implies an anti-empiricism that fails to chime with Laënnec's work, see Erwin H. Ackerknecht, *Medicine at the Paris Hospital, 1794–1848* (Baltimore, MD: Johns Hopkins Press, 1967), pp. 76, 198. See also George Rosen, 'Romantic Medicine: A Problem in Historical Periodization', *Bulletin of the History of Medicine*, 25.2 (1951), 149–58.

especially when they are deep and long lasting'].[19] The physiological shock of *passions tristes*, encompassing a range of emotions including grief, disappointed hope, and unrequited love, would depress the patient's vital energy and thus leave them susceptible to the wasting effects of consumption.[20]

Laënnec refers at length to a Parisian convent whose members all suffered from consumption due to the austere lifestyle imposed upon them: although their diet was normal for cloistered communities, 'l'esprit dans lequel on dirigeait ces religieuses produisait des effets aussi fâcheux que surprenans' ['The spirit in which these nuns were guided produced effects as unfortunate as they were surprising'].[21] He states that not only were the nuns forced to '[fixer] habituellement leur attention sur les vérités les plus terribles de la religion, mais on s'attachait à les éprouver par toutes sortes de contrariétés, afin de les faire parvenir dans le plus court espace de temps à un entier renoncement à leur propre volonté' ['habitually [fasten] their attention on the most terrible truths of religion, but it was undertaken to test them by all kinds of annoyances, in order to bring them in the shortest space of time to a complete renunciation of their own will'].[22] These conditions produced the same effect in all the community's members: after one or two months they would suffer from amenorrhea, an absence of menstruation, after which phthisis would take hold. Moreover, the sisters who left the order were cured, but that those who remained would eventually succumb to the disease.[23] Noting that the only survivors were the mother superior and the sisters who worked routinely in the kitchens and gardens, Laënnec remarks that they had the greatest opportunity to escape the rigours of the religious community, whereas the others 'paraissaient également devoir l'origine de leur maladie à des chagrins profonds et de longue durée' ['seemed to owe the origin of their illness to a deep and long-lasting grief'] that were unbroken by regular labour.[24] In short, then, although Laënnec understood consumption as an internal illness, he foregrounded how the disease could take hold due to unfavourable living situations that restricted free movement and provoked a general depression of spirits.

There are no indications in *Lamiel* that the eponymous heroine suffers from the *passions tristes* outlined by Laënnec: she endures no broken heart, no unrequited love, no emotional shock. Nevertheless, the Duchesse's castle has much in common with the Parisian convent to which Laënnec refers. Scholars observe that Lamiel's arrival at the castle is tantamount to her entry into a range of interdictions that limit her ability to move freely: Naomi Schor characterizes this version

[19] René-Théophile-Hyacinthe, *Traité de l'auscultation médiate et des maladies des poumons et du cœur*, 2 vols (Paris: J.-S. Chaudé, 1826), I, p. 646.

[20] See Frank M. Snowden, *Epidemics and Society: From the Black Death to the Present* (New Haven, CT: Yale University Press, 2019), p. 279.

[21] Laënnec, *Traité de l'auscultation médiate*, I, p. 647.

[22] Ibid, I, p. 647.

[23] Ibid., I, p. 647.

[24] Ibid., I, p. 648.

of the novel as driven by the progressive 'binding of female energy'.[25] Scott sees Lamiel in both substantial versions of the manuscript as a 'movement-hungry child', oppressed by the constraints on her physical freedom incurred at the castle.[26] These rules include the Duchesse's interdiction against walking quickly on the beautiful carpet in Lamiel's room; running in the garden; and the general rule that 'tout devait se faire lentement' ['everything had to be done slowly'].[27] These strict regulations crush the spirit of the eponymous heroine who becomes a 'gazelle enchaînée' ['chained gazelle'].[28] Beyond the physical limitations that these rules represent, they also affect Lamiel's spirits: as she is about to enter the castle, her adoptive mother tells her that the conditions will be so miserable that she will be happy to leave in a few months' time. The narrator notes that these words 'furent fatals pour Lamiel' ['were fatal for Lamiel'] and that 'tout son bonheur disparut à l'instant' ['all of her happiness disappeared in an instant'].[29] Fulfilling this prophecy, Lamiel is later described as 'pénétrée d'un profond découragement' ['filled with a profound despondency'] when she sees the serious demeanour of the older women with whom she will live, and after three days becomes so unhappy that she loses her appetite.[30]

After Lamiel fails to abide by the Duchesse's original interdictions, even more severe ones are put in place to curb her freedom: 'il fut décidé que Lamiel ne pourrait se promener, même dans le parterre, que dans la compagnie d'une des femmes de chambre de Madame, et ces demoiselles trouvaient toujours qu'il faisait trop humide, ou trop chaud, ou trop froid pour se promener' ['it was decided that Lamiel could only walk, even among the flowerbeds, in the company of one of Madame's chambermaids, and these ladies always found it too humid, or too hot, or too cold to walk'].[31] As in Laënnec's analysis of the cloistered sisters, the relative physical comfort is not enough to prevent an onset of consumption. Whilst examining Lamiel, Sansfin thinks to himself that his patient is ill 'malgré le commerce de la duchesse, l'excellent cuisinier, les primeurs, les beaux meubles du château, etc. etc.' ['despite the company of the duchess, the excellent cooking, the early seasonal vegetables, the castle's beautiful furniture, et cetera et cetera'], demonstrating that relative luxury is no antidote to the effects of imprisonment.[32] The restrictions imposed on Lamiel eventually cause so much physical suffering that she almost loses the desire to move around: 'Lamiel n'avait presque plus l'envie de se promener' ['Lamiel hardly had the desire to go for a walk anymore'].[33] She

[25] Schor, *Breaking the Chain*, p. 142.
[26] Scott, *Stendhal's Less-Loved Heroines*, p. 90.
[27] *ORC*, III, p. 1000.
[28] Ibid., III, p. 845.
[29] Ibid., III, p. 1000.
[30] Ibid., III, p. 1000.
[31] Ibid., III, p. 1000.
[32] Ibid., III, p. 1004.
[33] Ibid., III, p. 1001.

slowly descends into despair, 'toute la gaieté de la jeunesse avait disparu chez la jeune paysanne' ['all the cheerfulness of youth had disappeared from the young peasant girl'], which culminates in her serious illness.[34]

The eponymous heroine's situation conforms to other *causes occasionnelles* identified by Laënnec, such as overwork.[35] Sansfin blames Lamiel's consumption on being overworked as the Duchesse's *lectrice*: 'Cette jeune poitrine [...] a été enflammée pour longtemps et, peut-être, complètement perdue par les excès de lecture' ['These young lungs [...] had been inflamed for a long time, and are perhaps completely lost due to an excess of reading'].[36] Earlier in the novel, Lamiel's schoolmaster tries to prevent her from working for the Duchesse on the basis of her consumptive state, the teacher is 'effrayé du terrible message dont on l'avait chargé [...] annonça que, toute réflexion faite, Lamiel avait la poitrine trop délicate pour pouvoir accepter l'honneur que Madame la duchesse avait voulu lui faire' ['frightened by the terrible message with which he was charged [...] announced that, all things considered, Lamiel had a chest that was too delicate to accept the honour that Madame la Duchesse had bestowed upon her'].[37] In addition, according to Laënnec, consumption was rarely found in rural and coastal Normandy and Brittany.[38] Fittingly, then, Sansfin pronounces that 'voici un cas bien rare en *Normandie*' ['here is a case that is rare for *Normandy*'].[39] At repeated instances, then, the text shows us that Lamiel is ill and is thus a patient of Sansfin. However, as the rest of this chapter demonstrates, the metaphorical richness of the doctor–patient encounter points undermines the conventional hierarchy of the doctor–patient relationship. In its extraordinary doctor–patient encounter, wherein Sansfin convinces Lamiel to simulate severe symptoms of tuberculosis, the novel forges a new mould for the representation of nineteenth-century female patienthood.

Doctors, Fathers, and Dead Birds

After Lamiel has begun working in the castle as *lectrice*, Sansfin makes a remarkable proposal. Once a week he will behead a small bird and soak a sponge with

[34] Ibid., III, p. 1003. The nefarious effect of the Duchesse's castle on Lamiel contrasts the personal freedom afforded to Julien by prison in *Le Rouge et Le Noir* and to Fabrice by the titular charterhouse in *La Chartreuse de Parme*: Victor Brombert argues, for example, that Fabrice's retreat into a secluded religious community affords him personal liberation thanks to the severance with the outside world. See Victor Brombert, *Stendhal: Fiction and the Themes of Freedom* (Chicago, IL: University of Chicago Press, 1976), pp. 169–70.

[35] Laënnec, *De l'auscultation médiate*, I, pp. 94, 200, 205, 360, 453.

[36] *ORC*, III, p. 1015. Frank M. Snowden also mentions overwork as an important factor according to Laënnec. See Snowden, *Epidemics and Society*, p. 179.

[37] *ORC*, III, p. 998.

[38] Laënnec, *De l'auscultation médiate*, I, pp. 643–4.

[39] *ORC*, III, p. 1004; original emphasis.

its blood for Lamiel to use to simulate haemoptysis, the coughing up of bloodied sputum synonymous with tuberculosis from which Lamiel suffers only slightly. He says:

> Je veux [...] que vous consentiez à un meurtre horrible: tous les huit jours, je vous apporterai dans la poche de ma veste de chausse de Staub (le tailleur à la mode) un oiseau vivant. Je lui couperai la tête. Vous verserez le sang sur une petite éponge que vous placerez dans votre bouche. Aurez-vous ce courage? Pour moi, j'en doute. [...] Après, [...] dans les moments que vous passez auprès de la duchesse, de temps à autre vous cracherez le sang. Votre poitrine attaquée à ce point, on n'aura plus d'objection à tout ce que je voudrai faire faire pour vous amuser. Je vous l'ai déjà dit: votre maladie conduit au marasme; rien n'est plus dangereux chez les filles de votre âge. Mais, au fond, votre maladie n'était que de l'ennui.[40]

> I want [...] you to consent to a horrible murder: every week, I will bring you in the pocket of my jacket from Staub (the fashionable tailor of the day) a living bird. I will cut off its head. You will pour the blood onto a small sponge that you will place in your mouth. Will you be brave enough? For me, I doubt it. [...] Afterwards, [...] in the moments that you spend with the Duchesse, every now and then you will cough up the blood. Your lungs under attack to this extent, no one will object to anything I want to do for your enjoyment. I have already told you: your illness leads to stagnation; nothing is more dangerous in girls of your age. But, deep down, your illness was nothing but ennui.

On a narrative level, the reason for Sansfin's suggestion is clear. He believes that, by worsening the appearance of Lamiel's consumption, he can both dominate his patient and guarantee that the Duchesse will require his services more frequently, thus allowing him to exploit his patient for his own political ambitions. Despite the doctor's unorthodox approach, his proposed 'meurtre horrible', this *fausse phtisie* scene has been largely overlooked by scholars. Yet this episode has a transformative effect on the novel: indeed, in a note from 14 March 1841, Stendhal remarks that 'Un événement singulier change tous les rapports de Sansfin and Lamiel' ['A singular event changes the relationship between Sansfin and Lamiel completely'].[41] At stake in this dramatic performance, then, is the nature of the medical relationship in *Lamiel*. I argue that the potential of the scene's metaphorical signification demands that greater critical attention be paid to it: what does re-focalizing this scene from Lamiel's perspective reveal about what Sansfin, and many readers of the novel, perceive to be a conventionally hierarchical doctor–patient relationship?

[40] *ORC*, III, p. 1013.
[41] Ibid., III, p. 1083.

Laënnec characterizes haemoptysis, the production of bloodied sputum, as the most widely recognized sign of tuberculosis amongst the medical and general population: 'L'hémoptysie est communément regardée comme une des causes les plus fréquentes de la phthisie pulmonaire. [...] L'opinion vulgaire à cet égard n'est encore appuyée que sur une application peu réfléchie de l'axiome *post hoc, ergo propter hoc*' ['Haemoptysis is widely regarded as one of the most common causes of phthisis of the lungs. [...] The popular opinion in this regard is still based only on the thoughtless application of the axiom *post hoc, ergo propter hoc*'].[42] It is this sign of tuberculosis, the violent coughing up of blood in the later stages of the disease, that Sansfin and Lamiel choose to stage in the *fausse phtisie* scene. I argue here that the meaning of this performance is concealed in the iconography and metaphor of the medical encounter which in turn shines new light on the Stendhalian doctor–patient relationship.

The most striking element of the doctor–patient encounter in *Lamiel* is the murder of a small bird and Lamiel's placement of its blood in her mouth, equal parts symbolically allusive and sexually suggestive. The symbolism of birds in the visual iconography of nineteenth-century France was richly eroticized, an inheritance from Golden Age Dutch painting in which birds were often used as a euphemistic representation of the phallus.[43] However, by the eighteenth century this visual language had become less explicit, and birds instead operated as love tokens. In this new role, Elise Goodman argues that they tended to represent female virginity through their sexualized allusiveness and delicateness.[44] The most recognizable examples of a bird used to symbolize virginity are Jean-Baptiste Greuze's three *jeune fille* genre paintings that include a dead bird, exhibited in 1763, 1765, and 1800 respectively. Despite Greuze's diminishing fortunes after the turn of the century, the 1800 version entitled *L'Oiseau mort* was coolly reviewed in the *Coup d'œil sur le Salon de l'An VIII* as evidence of the artist's fall from fashion and the outdatedness of the dead bird trope, his artwork is evoked five times across Stendhal's writing.[45]

Greuze is mentioned in *Rome, Naples, et Florence*, in *Promenades dans Rome*, in *Histoire de la peinture en Italie* amongst a list of 'les artistes les plus célèbres', and in Stendhal's notes from the 1824 Salon.[46] Greuze makes a noteworthy appearance in *Voyage dans le midi de la France*, in which Stendhal describes a picturesque

[42] Laënnec, *De l'auscultation médiate*, I, p. 645.

[43] Kevin Chua, 'Dead Birds, or the Miseducation of the Greuze Girl', in *Performing the 'Everyday': The Culture of Genre in the Eighteenth Century*, ed. by Alden Cavanaugh (Newark, DE: University of Delaware Press, 2007), pp. 75–91 (p. 78); Elaine Shefer, 'The "Bird in the Cage" in the History of Sexuality: Sir John Everett Millais and William Holman Hunt', *Journal of the History of Sexuality*, 1.3 (1991), 446–80 (pp. 447–8).

[44] Elise Goodman, '"Les Jeux innocents": French Rococo Birding and Fishing Scenes', *Simiolus: Netherlands Quarterly for the History of Art*, 23.4 (1995), 251–67 (p. 251).

[45] Anita Brookner, *Greuze: The Rise and Fall of an Eighteenth-Century Phenomenon* (London: Elek, 1972), pp. 86–7.

[46] Stendhal, *Voyages en Italie*, ed. by Victor Del Litto (Paris: Gallimard, 2002), p. 459.

scene of a young boy sleeping. The passage recreates Greuze's atmospheric studies to render an intriguing encounter that took place whilst walking in Marseille in 1805, the same year as Greuze's death:

> Je trouvai, à côté de la porte, un joli enfant de quatre ans, qui dormait dans la position des enfants Jésus de Raphaël. Il avait une figure de Greuze, à cause de ses beaux yeux noirs et de ses cheveux blonds, tombant à grosses boucles sur ses épaules. Je le lui fis voir, elle le trouva charmant. Mais elle remarqua que ce sommeil avait une physionomie particulière: le visage et surtout la pose exprimaient un repos serein et tranquille; les yeux exprimaient la douleur. Nous demandâmes: on venait de lui raccommoder la jambe qu'il s'était cassée deux heures auparavant.[47]
>
> I found, by the door, a pretty child of four years old sleeping in the pose of Raphaël's children of Jesus. His beautiful dark eyes and blond hair falling in great curls across his shoulders gave him the air of a Greuze painting. I showed him to her, and she found him charming. But she noticed that his sleep had a particular physiognomy. The face, and especially the pose, expressed a serene and peaceful rest, while the eyes expressed pain. We asked him: his leg, which he had broken two hours before, had just been mended.

Here Stendhal explicitly refers to Greuze's work in order to evoke the quintessentially desolate atmosphere of paintings featuring melancholic-looking young boys such as *Le Petit Paresseux* from 1755, *Jeune garçon avec son livre de classe* from 1757, or *Tête de jeune garçon* from 1763, to name but a few. Stendhal's literary interest in the eighteenth century is well known: Kara Rabbitt outlines that Stendhal relies on eighteenth-century tropes to express how Lamiel, like Madame de Merteuil in *Les Liaisons dangereuses*, writes her freedom into existence throughout the novel.[48] My argument builds on these observations, but argues that the novel relies on, and subverts, eighteenth-century visual iconography as well as literary intertexts.

The most important and well-known of Greuze's three *jeune fille* genre paintings that include a dead bird is his 1765 *Jeune fille qui pleure son oiseau mort*, contemporaneously known as *La Pleureuse*. The painting depicts a melancholic young girl

[47] Stendhal, *Voyages en France*, ed. by Victor Del Litto (Paris: Gallimard, 1992), p. 791.

[48] Kara M. Rabbitt, 'L'Enfant libertine: pouvoir discursif et volonté narrative dans *Lamiel* de Stendhal', *Nineteenth Century French Studies*, 31.1 (2002), 66–83 (p. 78). Schor asserts that *Lamiel I* evokes the spirit of female freedom often found in the eighteenth century; *Lamiel II*, she argues, represents the eponymous heroine's insertion into the nineteenth-century world of female subordination and political marginalization. See Schor, *Breaking the Chain*, pp. 136, 142–5. Focusing on Sansfin's quasi-libertine education of Lamiel, Thompson compares him with the Marquis de Sade. See Thompson, *Lamiel, fille du feu*, pp. 91–4. For contrasting readings of the influence of Rousseau's *Émile* on *Lamiel* see Ansel, *Stendhal littéral*, p. 124; and Philippe Berthier, *Lamiel, ou, La Boîte de Pandore* (Paris: Presses universitaires de France, 1994), p. 30.

with blond curled hair and blushed cheeks. Her eyes shut, she holds her head in her left hand, and looks forlornly towards the bottom edge of the frame to the limp body of a dead yellow canary lying atop its opened cage. *La Pleureuse* is the most famous of the trio of dead bird paintings thanks to Denis Diderot's commentary on the 1765 Salon which included Greuze's painting. In this ekphrastic description, Diderot suggests that the dead bird should be understood as an allegory of lost virginity. Instead, he argues, the girl is crying about 'autre chose' ['something else'] than the bird itself:

> Le sujet de ce petit poème est si fin, que beaucoup de personnes ne l'ont pas entendu; ils ont cru que cette jeune fille ne pleurait que son serin. Greuze a déjà peint une fois le même sujet [*Le Miroir cassé*, 1763]. [...] Ne pensez-vous qu'il y aurait autant de bêtise à attribuer les pleurs de la jeune fille de ce Salon à la perte d'un oiseau, que la mélancolie de la jeune fille du Salon précèdent à son miroir cassé? Cet enfant pleure autre chose, vous dis-je. D'abord vous l'avez entendue, elle en convient; et son affliction le dit de reste. Cette douleur! à son âge! et pour un oiseau!—Mais quel âge a-t-elle donc?[49]

> The subject of this little ode is so subtle that many people have not understood it; they believed that the little girl was only crying for her canary. Greuze has already painted the same subject once [*The Broken Mirror*, 1763]. [...] Do you not think that there would be just as idiotic to attribute the tears of the young girl of this Salon to the loss of a bird, as the melancholy of the young girl of the most recent Salon to her broken mirror? This child is crying for something else, I tell you. First you understood her, and she suited this interpretation; her affliction says the rest. This pain! At her age! And for a bird! But how old is she?

Diderot's association between dead birds and lost female virginity echoes scholars' observations of the asymmetric power dynamic between doctor and patient in *Lamiel*: Michel Crouzet, for example, refers to the 'domptage de Lamiel' ['the taming of Lamiel'] by Sansfin.[50] Philippe Berthier characterizes the scene as emblematic of the doctor's consolidation of his power over Lamiel: 'Jamais Sansfin n'a davantage "possédé" Lamiel [...] qu'en ce moment où, dans le meurtre, elle accepte le sacrement maudit des initiés' ['Never had Sansfin better "possessed" Lamiel than in this moment when, during the murder, she accepts the cursed sacrament of the initiated'].[51] Such analyses are underpinned by the violence of the scene, notably the bird's summary execution by Sansfin and the violation of

[49] Denis Diderot, *Salons* (Paris: Gallimard, 2008), p. 136.
[50] Michel Crouzet, 'Le Dépucelage de Lamiel', in *Amicitia scriptor: littérature, histoire des idées, philosophie. Mélanges offerts à Robert Mauzi*, ed. by Annie Becq, Charles Porset and Alain Mothu (Paris: Champion, 1998), pp. 293–313 (p. 302).
[51] Berthier, *Lamiel, ou, La Boîte de Pandore*, p. 53.

Lamiel's body by forcing her to place the bird's blood inside her mouth. That birds were used in turn-of-the-century painting to depict female virginity deepens the parallels between this scene and a violent deflowering of the eponymous heroine, to say nothing of the motif of blood commonly associated with a broken hymen. Indeed, there is textual evidence that Stendhal saw a similar intention in Sansfin: in a plan dated 25 May 1840, Stendhal sketches how Sansfin intends to take Lamiel's virginity as part of his ploy, that 'le docteur veut prendre ce pucelage' ['the doctor wants to take her virginity'].[52]

However, that Sansfin *wants* to take Lamiel's virginity does not necessarily mean that this scene enacts his sordid fantasy. Instead, the iconography of the scene points towards a more complex metaphorical meaning that, in turn, reveals that Sansfin's corporeal desires are thwarted by Lamiel and that the medical authority of the doctor can be resisted through these metaphors. Recent scholarship on *La Pleureuse* has diverged from Diderot's allegorical reading of lost virginity, extending Anita Brookner's observation that Greuze's paintings always depict more than moralizing tropes since he 'cannot refrain from exploring, hinting, exposing' sexuality, and not just immorality, in his paintings.[53] Of course, Diderot admits that few contemporary observers of *La Pleureuse* understood the painting as an allegory of lost virginity, writing that 'le sujet de ce petit poème est si fin que beaucoup de personnes ne l'ont pas entendu'.[54] By examining how most contemporaries responded to the painting, Emma Barker argues that it was generally interpreted as an allegorization of the loss of childhood innocence engendered when a young girl acquires greater sexual knowledge as she enters womanhood. Barker argues that, rather than being a moralizing allegory of lost female virginity, *La Pleureuse* dramatizes the *jeune fille*'s newfound vulnerability to seduction now that she has reaches the age of nubility.[55] The painting thus dramatizes the creation of the category of virginity at a certain age, as well as the potential crisis brought about if the sacred deposit of her virginity is spent out of wedlock.[56]

Bernadette Fort foregrounds how Diderot, despite initially styling himself as a benevolent *homme sensible*, inserts himself into the position of a lover or seducer, thus taking advantage of the young girl's sexual vulnerability and the

[52] *ORC*, III, p. 1072.

[53] Brookner, *Greuze*, p. 90.

[54] Diderot, *Salons*, p. 136.

[55] Emma Barker, 'Reading the Greuze Girl: The Daughter's Seduction', *Representations*, 117.1 (2012), 86–119 (p. 100).

[56] The young girl's vulnerability to seduction is a key structuring device of eighteenth-century novels. See Nancy K. Miller, *The Heroine's Text: Readings in the French and English Novel, 1722–1782* (New York: Columbia University Press, 1980), pp. 4–5, 96–100. Kevin Chua observes that the emotive draw of *La Pleureuse* lies in its inconclusiveness: the outcome of the scenario imagined by Diderot is left uncertain, reflecting how Greuze captures the moment in which the young girl's virginity, and sexual value, is in jeopardy. See Chua, 'Dead Birds, or the Miseducation of the Greuze Girl', p. 89.

high personal cost of her seduction.[57] As Barker persuasively argues, Greuze's painting 'colludes with [the male spectator's] desire to keep her for himself rather than hand him over to a young man as morality dictates'.[58] Diderot acknowledges his sexual interest in the girl whilst simultaneously declaring his adherence to the need to respect her innocence: 'On s'approcherait de cette main pour la baiser, si on ne respectait cette enfant et sa douleur' ['We would approach this hand to kiss it, if we did not respect this child and her pain'].[59] Diderot's apophasis that 'Je ne suis pas père' ['I am not a father'] only adds to the quasi-incestuous overtones of his review.[60] Greuze's painting and Diderot's review coincide with other representations of quasi-incestuous father–daughter relationships in late-eighteenth-century culture.[61] Tony Tanner evidences how, in *La Nouvelle Héloïse*, Saint-Preux's allusion to incest in letter V, 'Je frémirais de porter la main sur tes chastes attraits plus que du plus vil inceste, et tu n'es pas dans une sûreté plus inviolable avec ton père qu'avec ton amant' ['I would shudder to lay my hand on your chaste attractions more than the vilest incest, and you are no more inviolable with your father than with your lover'], casts a long shadow over the text, amplifying the incestuous tones of a later scene in which Julie's father, angered by the thought of Saint-Preux as a son-in-law, physically assaults her.[62] From the iconography of dead birds in eighteenth-century painting, in addition to the ubiquity of representations of father–daughter incest, *La Pleureuse* can be seen to intradiegetically dramatize the precarious entrance of the *jeune fille* into the sexual marketplace. Through responses to the painting, such as Diderot's review, it intersects extradiegetically with a broader trend of the portrayal of incestuous father–daughter relationships in the late eighteenth century.

In *Lamiel*, the category of *jeune fille* is also associated with predatory relationships, a dynamic that is projected onto the doctor–patient relationship. For example, when speaking about Sansfin, the Abbé Clément believes that he is 'capable de tout afin de faire oublier sa bosse aux jeunes filles qu'il avait l'impertinence de courtiser' ['capable of anything to make the young girls, whom he had the impertinence to court, forget his hunchback'].[63] The doctor's interest in *jeunes filles* is evidenced fifty pages after the *fausse phtisie* scene. When Sansfin fears that the

[57] Bernadette Fort, 'The Greuze Girl: The Invention of a Pictorial Paradigm', *Studies in the History of Art*, 72 (2008), 128–51.

[58] Barker, 'Reading the Greuze Girl', p. 103.

[59] Diderot, *Salons*, p. 133.

[60] Ibid., p. 134.

[61] Barker, 'Reading the Greuze Girl', p. 107; Ellen Pollak, *Incest and the English Novel, 1684–1814* (Baltimore, MD: Johns Hopkins University Press, 2003), pp. 2–17.

[62] Jean-Jacques Rousseau, *La Nouvelle Héloïse. Théâtre. Poésies. Essais littéraires*, ed. by Bernard Gagnebin and Marcel Raymond, in Jean-Jacques Rousseau, *Œuvres complètes*, 5 vols, (Paris: Gallimard, 2012), II, p. 42. Tony Tanner, *Adultery in the Novel: Contract and Transgression* (Baltimore, MD: Johns Hopkins University Press, 1981), p. 114.

[63] *ORC*, III, pp. 973–4.

Abbé Clément's influence over Lamiel is increasing, the doctor tries to turn her against the older women who preoccupy themselves with moral codes:

> Combien de jeunes filles ne meurent pas avant vingt-trois ans [...] et alors à quoi bon toutes les gênes qu'elles se sont imposées depuis quinze ans, tous les plaisirs dont elles se sont privées pour gagner la bonne opinion de huit ou dix vieilles femmes formant la haute société du village?[64]

> How many young girls do not die before twenty-three years old [...] and so what good is all the discomfort they have imposed upon themselves since the age of fifteen, all the pleasures of which they have deprived themselves to win the good opinion of eight or ten old women that formed village's high society?

Here Sansfin echoes the legal and medical interest in the ages of fifteen (the average age for the onset of menses at the time) and sixteen (the age at which girls could marry).[65] There was a transition from the use of 'jeune fille' as a legal term in the eighteenth century to a medical one in the nineteenth century. In the 1762 edition of the *Dictionnaire de l'Académie française*, puberty is merely a juridical category, it is 'l'âge auquel la Loi permet de se marier' ['the age at which the law permits marriage'], noting that the age of puberty was fourteen for boys and twelve for girls.[66] In the 1835 edition, this legal definition gave way to a medical one: puberty became 'l'état des garçons et des filles qui sont nubiles' ['the state of girls and boys who are nubile'].[67] The changing meaning of *nubile* is also significant: the 1762 edition of the *Dictionnaire* notes that the category is only used to refer to girls; in 1835 the dictionary specifies that 'il se dit principalement des jeunes filles' ['principally used with reference to young girls'], suggesting the extent to which the category of *jeune fille* had become coterminous with physiological pubescence by the early nineteenth century.

With an increasingly menacing tone, Sansfin then attempts to persuade Lamiel to embrace a life of pleasure and gratification by enumerating the benefits to be gained:

> Il y a donc doublement à gagner à écouter la voix de la nature et à suivre tous ses caprices: d'abord l'on se donne du plaisir, ce qui est le seul objet pour lequel la race humaine est placée ici-bas; en second lieu, l'âme fortifiée par le plaisir, qui est son élément véritable, a le courage de n'omettre aucune des petites comédies

[64] *ORC*, III, p. 1023.

[65] For the average age of the onset of menses in the nineteenth century, see Edward Shorter, 'L'Âge des premières règles en France', *Annales*, 36.3 (1981), 495–511.

[66] *Le Dictionnaire de l'Académie française* (Paris: Bernard Brunet, 1762), p. 494, s.v. 'puberté'.

[67] *Le Dictionnaire de l'Académie française* (Paris: Firmin Didot frères, 1835), p. 528, s.v. 'puberté'.

nécessaires à une jeune fille pour gagner la bonne opinion des vieilles femmes en crédit dans le village.[68]

There is, therefore, doubly to be gained from listening to the voice of nature and following all of its whims: first, you give yourself to pleasure, which is the only object for which the human race is placed on this earth; second, the soul now fortified with pleasure, its true element, has the courage not to omit any of the little farces necessary for a young girl to win the good opinion of the old women of credit in the village.

Sansfin models himself on a Diderotesque *homme sensible*, claiming to be acting in the female subject's interests but simultaneously concealing a malevolent ulterior motive. By accusing older women of policing the personal and sexual freedom of *jeunes filles*, Sansfin attempts to dissimulate the tyranny of his own quasi-paternal power through his representation of maternal authority as the true brake on Lamiel's personal freedom.[69] Lamiel's status as a *jeune fille* is thus marked by the doctor's increased quasi-incestuous sexual interest in her.

As we saw in Chapter One, the so-called natural authority of doctors and fathers are indelibly connected to one another. In the medical humanities, Hans-Georg Gadamer compares the doctor–patient relationship to other 'fundamentally unequal' relationships such as that between father and daughter, and re-readings of paternal desires in *La Pleureuse* elucidate not only the asymmetric relationship between Lamiel and Sansfin but also how this inequality derives from the quasi-incestuous overtones of the scene.[70] Although Lamiel's biological father is absent from the novel, she experiences no shortage of quasi-paternal figures including M. Hautemare, Sansfin, and the Abbé Clément, who attempt to dominate her by shaping her in their own image. Berthier observes the quasi-incestuous tone of the doctor–patient encounter, seeing the bird as a synecdoche of Lamiel: 'c'est Lamiel bien sûr, beaucoup plus que l'oiseau, qui se voit immolée, victimisée, consommée par un sacrificateur qui est aussi un père puisque, ne l'oublions pas, elle est aussi la "fille" de ce Maître incestueux' ['it is Lamiel, of course, much more than the bird, who sees herself immolated, victimized, consumed by a high priest who is also a father since, let us not forget, she is also the "daughter" of this incestuous master'].[71] Indeed, Sansfin's desire to deflower Lamiel, to 'prendre ce pucelage' ['take this virginity'], intersects with his paternalistic feeling

[68] *ORC*, III, p. 1023.

[69] Sansfin's insinuation echoes other over-bearing Stendhalian mothers. For the importance of the maternal in *Le Rouge et le Noir*, and Julien's misguided preoccupation with paternalistic power, see Naomi Segal, *The Adulteress's Child: Authorship and Desire in the Nineteenth-Century Novel* (Cambridge: Polity Press, 1992), p. 63.

[70] Hans-Georg Gadamer, *The Enigma of Health: The Art of Healing in a Scientific Age* (Stanford, CA: Stanford University Press, 1996), p. 113.

[71] Berthier, *Lamiel, ou, La Boîte de Pandore*, p. 53.

towards her. For example, when he first describes Lamiel's consumptive condition to the Duchesse, he refers to her as 'cette aimable enfant' ['this lovely child'].[72] Sansfin's famous declaration, that '[Lamiel] sera à moi' ['[Lamiel] will be mine'] can thus be read in light of the previous discussion of the sexual status of the *jeune fille*.[73] On the one hand, Sansfin may wish to possess her in a predatorily sexual way; on the other hand, the fact that he feels as if Lamiel should belong to him evokes the asymmetric, and frequently eroticized, father–daughter relationship witnessed in Greuze's *La Pleureuse* and Diderot's review. The covert paternal-sexual desires in *La Pleureuse* elucidate not only the asymmetric doctor–patient relationship between Lamiel and Sansfin but also how this inequality derives from the quasi-incestuous overtones of the scene. The *fausse phtisie* scene, for all its iconographical and metaphorical meaning, boils down to the asymmetric relationship between doctor and patient.

The subjugation of Lamiel to her doctor's will therefore seems to be almost certain. Yet, the specificity of the doctor–patient encounter in fact undermines this conventionally hierarchical power dynamic between doctor and patient. The deliberateness and centrality of the bird's summary execution in *Lamiel* is dramatically violent, particularly so given that *La Pleureuse* does not narrativize how the bird died, and Diderot insinuates that it was a passive demise occurring from neglect (interpretable as the girl's 'neglect' to properly guard her virginity).[74] Echoing Diderot's comments, and operating within a heteronormative paradigm of sexual relations, Freud proposes that the loss of virginity inevitably 'not only binds a woman to a man but also "unleashes an archaic reaction of hostility against the man"'.[75] Kristeva argues that, following the woman's binding to a man through sexual relations that Freud outlines, 'Decapitation, which is a symbolic substitute for castration, thus appears as vengeance against the loss of virginity'.[76] Although we have seen that the iconography of dead birds and young girls goes beyond a straightforward allegorization of lost virginity, Kristeva's observation highlights the symbolic violence of the act of execution. Seen from this perspective, the bird's symbolic execution is tantamount to Lamiel's destruction of the iconography invested with the essence of female sexual value on which *La Pleureuse* relies. Stendhal's novel thus stages the execution of the bird whose death causes the subject of Greuze's painting so much distress, refuting the eighteenth-century association between the bird motif with a young girl's sexual value. Lamiel's participation in the bird's execution challenges Ansel's assertion that although Lamiel refuses marriage, 'cela ne saurait suffire à en faire une

[72] *ORC*, III, p. 1004.
[73] Ibid., III, p. 1115.
[74] Diderot, *Salons*, p. 134.
[75] Cited in Julia Kristeva, *The Severed Head: Capital Visions*, trans. by Jody Gladding (New York: Columbia University Press, 2014), p. 78.
[76] Ibid., p. 78.

féministe consciente des handicaps liés à sa condition de femme' ['this would not be enough to make her a feminist aware of the handicaps linked to her condition as a woman'].[77]

Although the execution is Sansfin's idea, and the doctor goes as far as to characterize the *fausse phtisie* ruse as the application of 'la terreur' ['terror'], Lamiel's participation in the bird's summary execution in this extraordinary doctor–patient encounter constitutes an attack on quasi-paternal power.[78] All forms of paternal authority were deemed to be in crisis following the Revolution of 1789: for example, Lynn Hunt reads decapitation as a violent act intended to dislodge tyrannical paternal power, originating from the guillotining of Louis XVI in 1793.[79] Peter Brooks argues that, in *Le Rouge et le Noir*, paternity is 'an issue of obsessive importance' for Stendhal's protagonists, reflecting the century's political turbulence and seemingly chaotic search for a national quasi-paternal figure.[80] As mentioned previously, Sansfin is but one in a chain of father figures who seek to dominate Lamiel, imitating how, in *Le Rouge et le Noir*, 'Julien is set in relation to a series of ideal or possible fathers, but in a curious manner whereby each father figure claims authority, or has authority conferred on him, just at the moment when he is about to be replaced'.[81] The connection between Lamiel and Julien, forged through their relationships to paternal figures, reflects Gérard Genette's argument that Stendhal's reader is 'conduit à d'incessantes comparaisons entre les situations, les personnages, les sentiments, les actions, dégageant instinctivement les correspondances par superposition et mise en perspective' ['led to make endless comparisons between situations, characters, feelings, actions, instinctively bringing out connections through superimposition and perspective'].[82]

The doctor–patient encounter in *Lamiel* thus marks both the highpoint, but also the inevitable downfall, of Sansfin's tyranny over Lamiel. The fact of Sansfin's own belief in Lamiel's subjugation betrays his ironic removal from influence since, after this scene, Sansfin becomes engaged in a protracted struggle with the Abbé Clément for control of Lamiel. Although Sansfin may believe himself to be in control of the bird's execution, and by default Lamiel herself, the recurrence of the execution motif points towards his doomed quasi-paternalistic power. The bird's summary execution recalls the destruction of tyrannical quasi-paternal power in

[77] Ansel, *Stendhal littéral*, p. 180. In the same vein, Scott challenges Ansel's argument that Lamiel is not a feminist because of her financial reliance on men, which he characterizes as tantamount to prostitution. See Scott, *Stendhal's Less-Loved Heroines*, p. 113, n. 34.

[78] *ORC*, III, p. 1015.

[79] Lynn Hunt, *The Family Romance of the French Revolution* (London: Routledge, 1992), pp. 17–52.

[80] Peter Brooks, 'The Novel and the Guillotine; or, Fathers and Sons in *Le Rouge et le Noir*', *PMLA*, 97.3 (1982), 348–62 (p. 348).

[81] Ibid., p. 352.

[82] Gérard Genette, *Figures II* (Paris: Seuil, 1979), p. 179. By contrast, Ansel argues that Lamiel 'n'est pas une sorte de Julien femelle' ['is not a sort of female Julien'] on account of her peasant upbringing and gender. See Ansel, *Stendhal littéral*, p. 138. Here I suggest that this focus on biographical details neglects the more important characteristics that Julien and Lamiel have in common.

other Stendhal novels, such as *Le Rouge et le Noir*: through the motif of execution the novel rejects not just Sansfin's specific brand of paternal tyranny but the model of paternal-medical authority itself. By subverting the iconography of dead birds and lost virginity, Lamiel's participation in the *fausse phtisie* scene demonstrates her resistance to these paradigms of control, including that of the hierarchical doctor–patient relationship.[83]

Lamiel's reaction to this symbol execution further indicates her subversion of the hierarchical doctor–patient relationship during this singular medical encounter. Whereas the intense distress of the young girl inspired by the canary's death is foregrounded by Greuze, Stendhal instead traces Lamiel's ambiguous reaction to the bird's execution. At first, Lamiel simulates a reaction similar to that of the subject of *La Pleureuse*, hiding her face in her handkerchief and experiencing a profound distress at the bird's death: 'La vue de la mort donnée à ce petit être fort gentil avait bouleversé profondément l'âme de la jeune fille' ['The sight of this gentle little creature's death had deeply shaken the soul of the young girl'].[84] Yet, Lamiel then becomes emboldened by her involvement in the subterfuge. Although she is disgusted by the sight of blood, Lamiel also experiences the sensation of crime and deceit through her engagement in the ruse:

> Quoique le sang du pauvre petit oiseau [...] lui inspirât d'abord beaucoup de répugnance, cependant [Sansfin] parvint à lui faire placer dans la bouche la petite éponge imprégnée de sang, et de plus, ce qui valait bien mieux, par le ton de voix qu'il affecta, le docteur donna à Lamiel non pas la conviction, mais bien mieux la sensation qu'elle commettait un grand crime.[85]

> Although the blood of the poor little bird [...] initially horrified her, nevertheless [Sansfin] managed to make her place the small sponge soaked with blood in her mouth; what is more, by the tone of voice he used, the doctor gave Lamiel not the conviction but, even better, the feeling that she was committing a great crime.

In fact, Lamiel's role in the ruse is the culmination of her burgeoning interest in criminality. Twenty pages earlier, she discovers the criminal exploits of Mandrin and Cartouche after which she illicitly sells Monsieur Hautemare's copy of Virgil.[86] In the earlier manuscript, Lamiel's interest in Mandrin and Cartouche anticipates Lamiel's life with the fugitive Valbaire and Lamiel's eventual arson of the Palais de Justice in the version written in October–December 1839.[87] Lamiel's knowing participation in what Sansfin styles as a criminal murder reflects

[83] Brooks make a similar argument regarding the rejection of paternal authority in *Le Rouge et le Noir*. See Brooks, 'The Novel and the Guillotine', p. 360.
[84] *ORC*, III, p. 1015.
[85] Ibid., III, pp. 1014–15.
[86] Ibid., III, p. 993.
[87] Ibid., III, p. 954.

her growing interest in criminality and danger. Beauvoir argues that Stendhal's heroines achieve freedom through inner experiences such as Lamiel's reaction to the bird's murder: 'Ces femmes tout simplement sont *vivantes*; elles savent que la source des vraies valeurs n'est pas dans les choses extérieures, mais dans les cœurs' ['These women are quite simply *alive*; they know that the origin of true values is not in exterior things, but in their hearts'].[88] Lamiel's curious participation in the *fausse phtisie* scene, her willingness to place the bird's blood in her mouth, despite her initial disgust, is motivated by her underlying sense of freedom. As Beauvoir writes, 'La liberté de son esprit lui permet de reprendre à son compte tous les mouvements de sa curiosité' ['The freedom of her mind allows her to take over all the vagaries of her curiosity'].[89] Lamiel may imitate the subject of *La Pleureuse* to a certain extent, but inflects her reaction to the bird's murder with the delectable, and novel, sensation of having committed a crime, an aspect that refutes what Diderot calls the 'air rêveur et mélancolique' ['dreamlike, melancholic appearance'] of *La Pleureuse*.[90]

From this analysis, despite the episodic nature of Lamiel's encounter with Sansfin, the doctor–patient relationship emerges as one that initially appears in the novel as fundamentally asymmetric but that is overturned by the singular medical encounter that takes place between Lamiel and Sansfin. The incestuous overtones of Sansfin's authority over Lamiel are turned against him: Lamiel rejects not just his control, but the model of incestuous paternal authority in general. Visual imagery is central here: the manipulation of avian iconography and its link to female puberty demonstrates the extent to which the medical relationship is entangled in a web of other relationships and discourses.

Blood and Guts

Given the centrality of Lamiel's body to the success of this ruse, the scene doubtlessly relies on themes of corporeality and embodiment. In the medical humanities, themes connected to bodily fluids (such as blood, bile, or faeces) are an integral, although often taboo, element in understanding medicine. For example, scholars such as Alan Bleakley explore doctors' feelings of abjection and disgust when confronted with the ill or deformed body in order to tackle a perceived insensibility on the part of the medical professional.[91] These visceral fluids thus hinge on the doctor–patient relationship: the corporeality and hypervisibility of the patient's body, expressed through the appearance of bodily fluids that are

[88] Simone de Beauvoir, *Le Deuxième Sexe: les faits et les mythes*, 2 vols (Paris: Gallimard, 2012), I, p. 380.
[89] Ibid., I, p. 388.
[90] Diderot, *Salons*, p. 134.
[91] Alan Bleakley, *Educating Doctors' Senses through the Medical Humanities: 'How Do I Look?'* (Abingdon; New York: Routledge, 2020), pp. 27–38.

usually kept away from public view, contributes to the unique status of the medical relationship. In *Lamiel*, the violent coughing up of the bird's blood draws attention to the role and meaning of this vital fluid. Blood is often associated with the abject: Kristeva defines abjection as the feeling provoked when a given subject experiences their own corporeality. The discovery of the limit at which their 'self' meets the 'Other' threatens the integrity and sovereignty of the former: 'Il y a, dans l'abjection, une de ces violentes et obscures révoltes de l'être contre ce qui le menace et qui lui paraît venir d'un dehors ou d'un dedans exorbitant, jeté à côté du possible, du tolérable, du pensable' ['There is, in abjection, one of those violent and obscure revolts of the being against that which threatens it and that seems to come from an exorbitant outside or inside, thrown in with the possible, the tolerable, the thinkable'].[92] The subject's corporeality is primarily confronted through an encounter with a bodily fluid such as blood or faeces, or other repulsive material such as mud: 'Ces déchets chutent pour que je vive, jusqu'à ce que, de perte en perte, il ne m'en reste rien, et que mon corps tombe tout entier au-delà de la limite, *cadere*, cadavre' ['This rubbish falls away so that I can live, until, from loss to loss, I am left with nothing and my whole body falls beyond the limits, *cadere*, cadaver'].[93] Producing the terror of abjection is the primary aim of the *fausse phtisie* ruse: earlier in the novel the Duchesse is horrified when Sansfin suggests that Lamiel would begin coughing up blood owing to her neglect, suggesting that she would be 'mourante et pouvait à chaque instant être saisie d'un vomissement de sang pendant lequel elle serait morte dans [les] bras [de la Duchesse]' ['dying and could, at any moment, be seized with the vomiting of blood during which she would have died in [the] arms [of the Duchess]'].[94]

Other scholars observe the prevalence of abject materials in Stendhal's œuvre. Mud, according to Berthier, is 'une obsession chez Stendhal qui, d'un soin méticuleux et sourcilleux de l'impeccabilité de sa personne, ne redoute rien tant que de se voir maculé' ['an obsession for Stendhal, who, meticulous and careful with the impeccability of his person, fears nothing so much as to see himself stained'].[95] In *Lucien Leuwen*, Lucien is disgusted when he swallows some of the mud thrown at him by political protestors, 'La boue et les tronçons de choux volaient de tous côtés dans la calèche' ['Mud and pieces of cabbage flew everywhere around the carriage'], which Scott identifies as revealing to himself Lucien's own status as a subjective being.[96] At the Battle of Waterloo in *La Chartreuse de*

[92] Julia Kristeva, *Pouvoirs de l'horreur: essai sur l'abjection* (Paris: Seuil, 1980), p. 9. For Kristeva's call to divest the medical humanities from its concern with the opposition between the 'objectivity of science' and the 'subjectivity of culture', see Julia Kristeva, Marie Rose Moro, John Ødemark, and Eivind Engebretsen, 'Cultural Crossings of Care: An Appeal to the Medical Humanities', *Medical Humanities*, 44.1 (2018), 55–8.

[93] Kristeva, *Pouvoirs de l'horreur*, p. 11.

[94] *ORC*, III, p. 1007.

[95] Berthier, *Lamiel, ou, La Boîte de Pandore*, p. 43.

[96] Stendhal, *Œuvres romanesques complètes II*, ed. by Yves Ansel, Philippe Berthier, and Xavier Bourdenet, Bibliothèque de la Plèiade, 13, 3 vols (Paris: Gallimard, 2007), II, p. 496. Maria Scott, 'Stendhal's Muddy Realism', *Dix-Neuf*, 16.1 (2012), 15–27.

Parme, Fabrice fixates on icons of abjection: notably corpses and the mingling of blood with mud on the churned-up field: 'Ce qui le frappait surtout, c'était la saleté des pieds de ce cadavre qui déjà était dépouillé de ses souliers, et auquel on n'avait laissé qu'un mauvais pantalon tout souillé de sang' ['What particularly struck him was the dirtiness of corpse's feet, which had already been stripped of its boots, and which only had left on it a poor pair of trousers soaked with blood'].[97] And, later, the emphasis returns to the repulsion produced in Fabrice: 'Ce qui lui sembla horrible, ce fut un cheval tout sanglant qui se débattait sur la terre labourée, en engageant ses pieds dans ses propres entrailles; [...] le sang coulait dans la boue' ['What seemed horrible to him was a bloodied horse that was struggling on the churned-up land, placing its hooves on its own entrails; [...] blood flowed into the mud'].[98] In *Lamiel*, Sansfin falls into mud whilst arguing with a gaggle of local washerwomen:

> Ce mouvement brusque et sec opéra la séparation du docteur et de la selle; le docteur, qui se penchait en avant, tomba net dans le bourbier, la tête la première; la boue avait bien un demi-pied de profondeur, et le docteur n'eut d'autre mal que celui de la honte, mais cette honte fut entière.[99]

> This sudden, sharp movement effected the separation of the doctor from his saddle: the doctor, who was leaning forward, fell head first into the mud; but the mud was a good half-foot deep, and the doctor endured no harm other than shame, but that shame was extreme.

The leitmotif of abject materials in Stendhal's novels thus reveals the fragility of the protagonist's sense of self, either through a sense of disgust as for Lucien, horror for Fabrice, or shame for Sansfin.

Although Stendhalian heroes such as Lucien and Fabrice, and anti-heroes such as Sansfin, have in common their encounters with abject material, the interaction between the bird's blood and Lamiel is striking given the cultural association between blood and the female body.[100] According to Mary Douglas, the marginalization of the female body is justified by the supposed poisonous effect of feminine bodily fluids, even though the male body is equally viscous: 'Females are correctly seen as, literally, the entry by which the pure content may be adulterated. Males are treated as pores through which the precious stuff may ooze out and be lost, with the whole system being thereby enfeebled'.[101]

97 *ORC*, III, p. 176.
98 Ibid., III, p. 181.
99 Ibid., III, pp. 985–6. Berthier also comments that these muddy instances are parallels of one another; see Berthier, *Lamiel, ou, La Boîte de Pandore*, p. 43.
100 Kristeva, *Pouvoirs de l'horreur*, p. 20.
101 Mary Douglas, *Purity and Danger: An Analysis of the Concepts of Pollution and Taboo* (London; New York: Routledge, 2005), p. 127.

Similarly, Jean-Paul Sartre connects feminine viscosity with a threat to submerge the subject in a way that mirrors the threat posed to the self by abject materials, writing that 'c'est une activité molle, baveuse et féminine d'aspiration, il vit obscurément sous mes doigts et je sens comme un vertige, il m'attire en lui comme un fond d'un précipice pourrait m'attirer' ['it is a soft, slimy, and feminine action of sucking that lives obscurely under my fingers and that I sense like a dizziness; it draws me to it like a bottom of a precipice could draw me to itself'].[102]

The threatening feminine sexuality of these abject encounters is also pointed out by Stendhal scholars. Berthier characterizes Sansfin's fall into the mud as an 'éclaboussement sexuel parfaitement assouvissant pour lui' ['perfectly fulfilling sexual satisfaction for him'], highlighting a link between abject material and sexuality.[103] The presence of the gaggle of local washerwomen highlights this dimension of sexual fulfilment or, rather, humiliation that threatens the masculine sense of self. Regarding *Lucien Leuwen*, Scott links this fear of female sexual desire to Lucien's encounter with abjection: 'Sa peur en matière sexuelle serait ainsi, dans cette logique, entièrement en accord avec son affolement lorsque la foule à Blois lui jette de la boue à la figure' ['His fear in sexual matters would thus be, according to this logic, entirely in accordance with his panic when the crowd in Blois throws mud in his face'].[104] At the end of the first half of *Lucien Leuwen*, the eponymous hero is repulsed by the sight of the blood that Doctor Du Poirier smears over the front of his apron during an elaborately faked childbirth scene: '[Lucien] vit arriver dans l'antichambre le docteur essoufflé portant l'enfant dans un linge qui lui parut taché de sang' ['[Lucien] saw the breathless doctor arrive in the anteroom, carrying the child in a cloth that seemed to him to be stained with blood'].[105] The sight of blood, associated with illicit feminine sexuality through the presence of the infant that Du Poirier remarks must not be Lucien's, provokes sufficient horror in Lucien to almost force him to flee: 'Il fut sur le point de sortir de sa cachette et de s'enfuir' ['He was about to leave his hiding place and flee'].[106] We will return to this scene from *Lucien Leuwen* in more detail.

The blood-soaked sponge episode in *Lamiel*, however, is different from these earlier examples of abject encounters from Stendhal's œuvre. Whereas Lucien, Fabrice, and Sansfin all confront abject material by unfortunate accident, Lamiel actively agrees to placing the blood in her mouth as mentioned previously. Lamiel's consent is not easily given since she is afraid of the blood. Indeed, her initial disgust

[102] Jean-Paul Sartre, *L'Être et le néant: essai d'ontologie phénoménologique*, ed. by Arlette Elkaïm-Sartre (Paris: Gallimard, 1943), p. 655. See also Elizabeth Grosz, *Volatile Bodies: Toward a Corporeal Feminism* (Bloomington, IN: Indiana University Press, 1994), pp. 194–5.

[103] Berthier, *Lamiel, ou, La Boîte de Pandore*, p. 43.

[104] Maria Scott, 'Le Réalisme et la peur du désir? Le cas de *Lucien Leuwen*', *L'Année stendhalienne*, 9 (2010), p. 53.

[105] *ORC*, II, p. 354.

[106] Ibid., II, p. 355.

at the proposed ruse confirms the sensation of repulsion when faced with abject material, coinciding with the feeling that Kristeva identifies: 'Quoique le sang du pauvre petit oiseau que le docteur apporta à sa malade lui inspirât d'abord beaucoup de répugnance, cependant il parvint à lui faire placer dans la bouche la petite éponge imprégnée de sang' ['Although the blood of the poor little bird [...] initially horrified her, nevertheless [Sansfin] managed to make her place the small sponge soaked with blood in her mouth'].[107] Here, the use of the imperfect subjunctive draws attention to the fact that Lamiel has overcome her initial disgust: despite acknowledging the repulsiveness of the act, she nevertheless agrees to go through with the tuberculosis performance.[108] Sansfin also foregrounds the macabre nature of the act, referring to the ruse as a 'meurtre horrible' and detailing that, although he will decapitate the bird, it is Lamiel who must pour out its blood, soak a sponge with it, and then place the sponge in her mouth.[109] The doctor–patient encounter thus places Lamiel in direct contact with the repulsive material of the bird's blood and thereby produces the psychological threat to the self that Kristeva outlines. Rather than being subjected to abjection, as in the case of Lucien who is repulsed by the sight of blood that he believes to belong to Bathilde, by placing the bird's blood inside her mouth Lamiel embraces the abject. By embracing bodily fluids usually regarded as taboo, the novel appropriates discourse of the embodied patient and thus amplifies the inversion of the doctor–patient relationship elsewhere established through the use of avian iconography.

Moreover, Lamiel's participation in the *fausse phtisie* scene not only brings her in contact with a form of abject femininity but does so through performance and gesture, pointing towards how the doctor–patient relationship can be staged or manipulated even when visceral elements are included in that performance. Scholars have pointed out Lamiel's taste for performance: writing on the sources for *Lamiel*, Jean Prévost foregrounds that Lamiel's willingness to adopt disguises is 'l'un des génies de Lamiel; il est essentiel au personnage de l'amazone' ['one of the genius elements of Lamiel: it is essential to the character of the Amazon'].[110] Lamiel's participation in the ruse is tantamount to her willingness to play the role of a gravely ill consumptive patient. Lamiel challenges and changes the paradigms of desire, as Berthier remarks regarding her use of holly paste to make herself appear more ugly to male onlookers: 'C'est dans le geste même par lequel elle se rend non désirable, et nie sa féminité selon les canons invétérés de la parade sexuelle, qu'elle la pose le plus fortement dans sa dimension redéfinie de conquête et de choix, selon des critères librement fixes' ['It is in the very gesture by which she makes herself undesirable, and denies her femininity according to the inveterate

[107] *ORC*, III, pp. 1014–15.
[108] Ibid., III, p. 1015.
[109] Ibid., III, p. 1013.
[110] Jean Prévost, *Essai sur les sources de 'Lamiel': les amazones de Stendhal, le procès de Lacenaire* (Lyon: Imprimeries réunies, 1942), p. 17.

canons of the sexual parade, that she poses it most strongly in her redefined dimension of conquest and choice, according to criteria that is freely fixed'].[111] Because of medicine's presumption that patients truly suffer from the diseases with which they are diagnosed, the notion of Lamiel's performance of haemoptysis exposes and undoes medicine's implicit belief in the authenticity of disease. Moreover, by pretending to have more severe consumption symptoms than she does, Lamiel affirms her potential for living a reality different to the one within which she presently exists. As Scott observes, Lamiel's 'talent for daring self-transformation is closely linked to her self-affirmation.'[112] Lamiel is not the only female protagonist in Stendhal's œuvre with a passion for disguise. In *Mina de Vanghel* the eponymous heroine attempts to make herself more ugly: 'Chaque jour, Mina se levait de grand matin afin de pouvoir pendant deux heures se livrer aux soins de s'enlaidir' ['Every day, Mina would get up early in order to be able to spend two hours making herself ugly'].[113] Mina achieves this by resorting, like Lamiel, to a paste composed of holly: 'Une légère décoction de feuilles de houx, appliquée chaque matin sur ses mains délicates, leur donnait l'apparence d'une peau rude' ['A light concoction of holly leaves, applied each morning to her delicate hands, giving them an appearance of rough skin'].[114]

Agreeing to the ruse allows the terror Lamiel first experienced at the sight of the bird's blood to be inflicted upon the Duchesse since the sight of the blood convinces her to give Lamiel whatever she desires. Although Sansfin may believe that he has inflicted '*la terreur*' on Lamiel and the Duchesse, it is Lamiel who overcomes the horror of the abject and grows bolder because of her involvement in the tuberculosis performance.[115] Through the ironic self-Othering of the scene, Lamiel renders herself abject, heightening the sexual threat of her body, and dramatically performs her femininity. Although true emancipation may be impossible for Lamiel, by deliberately placing herself in close contact with feminine-coded abject material in this staged bedside encounter, Lamiel finds a degree of personal freedom within the otherwise hierarchical doctor–patient relationship.

Scholars often read Sansfin's resolve as the imposition of his will over Lamiel: Thompson, for example, mentions the 'viol symbolique par Sansfin que constitue l'épisode du oiseau' ['symbolic rape by Sansfin that the bird episode constitutes'].[116] However, drawing out the consensual aspects of Lamiel's performance foregrounds the extent to which the characterization of a conventionally hierarchical doctor–patient relationship between Lamiel and Sansfin can be revised.

[111] Berthier, *Lamiel, ou, La Boîte de Pandore*, p. 86.
[112] Maria Scott, 'Performing Desire: Stendhal's Theatrical Heroines', *French Studies*, 62.3 (2008), 259–70 (p. 265).
[113] *ORC*, I, p. 308.
[114] Ibid., I, p. 308.
[115] Ibid., III, p. 1015. Emphasis original.
[116] Crouzet, 'Le Dépucelage de Lamiel', p. 302. Thompson, *Lamiel, fille du feu*, p. 117.

In the scene, Lamiel in fact agrees to participate in Sansfin's ruse.[117] In an earlier version of the novel, Lamiel smears holly paste onto her face in order to deflect the leering gazes of young men. The guise is suggested to her by an apothecary, who asks a crowd of listeners whether their disgust at the paste will be enough to deter them from smearing it on their cheeks: 'Auriez-vous de la répugnance, dit-il en s'adressant plus particulièrement à Lamiel, à mettre une de ces feuilles pilées sur une de vos joues?' ['"Are you disgusted," he said, addressing Lamiel in particular, "at the thought of putting these pounded leaves on one of your cheeks?"'].[118] Defiantly, Lamiel chooses to nevertheless smear the unsightly paste onto her cheek, embracing the repulsive material and rejecting beauty as defined by the male gaze. Lamiel's contact with abject material through her participation in the *fausse phtisie* ruse is also consensual: Sansfin insists that Lamiel must agree to the ruse, 'Je veux que vous consentiez', which Lamiel does by laughing at the ruse and exclaiming that Sansfin is 'amusant' ['entertaining'], and subsequently assuming her role in the plot.[119] Lamiel's consent, although implicit, contrasts with other Stendhalian characters' accidental encounters with abject material, thus suggesting the singularity of her agreeing to the tuberculosis plot. For example, the encounters with abject material by heroes such as Julien and Fabrice, as well as the anti-hero Sansfin, are all by misfortune or unhappy coincidence. By contrast, in both the holly paste disguise and the *fausse phtisie* scene, Lamiel freely chooses to play the role offered to her by a medical man, especially when it involves close contact with repugnant fluids, reinforcing that her performance is a manifestation of her free will.

Lamiel's agreement to participating to the ruse is dependent on the outcome of both acts: the apothecary promises her that 'Tant que vous n'aurez pas lavé cette joue, vous serez laide, et pour peu que vous cachiez cette joue avec votre mouchoir, je vous jure qu'aucun de ces hâbleurs de commis voyageurs ne vous ennuiera de ses propos galants' ['Until you wash this cheek, you will be ugly, and as long as you hide this cheek with your handkerchief, I swear that none of those hackneyed travellers will bore you with their gallant words'], thus allowing Lamiel to reject the otherwise objectifying male gaze.[120] Later Lamiel applies the paste again to ward off the leering of young men at a Rouennais theatre, the setting drawing attention to the performative nature of Lamiel's gesture.[121] In the case of the *fausse phtisie* scene, Lamiel primarily gains knowledge of societal hypocrisy. Thanks to Sansfin's misanthropic explanation of the lies inherent in all speech acts, Lamiel gleefully realizes her own duplicity, adding excitement to

[117] Ansel, *Stendhal littéral*, pp. 32 and 123.
[118] *ORC*, III, p. 910. The apothecary's question mirrors Sansfin's asking whether Lamiel is brave enough to put the bloodied sponge in her mouth.
[119] Ibid., III, pp. 1013 and 1014.
[120] Ibid., III, p. 910.
[121] Ibid., III, p. 994.

banal speech acts: 'quand je dis qu'il y a trois lieues et demie d'ici à Avranches, je dis un mensonge! Ah! mon pauvre docteur, quelles sornettes vous me débitez!' ['when I say that there are three and a half leagues to Avranches from here, I'm lying! Oh, my poor doctor, what nonsense you are telling me!'].[122] From this point on, Lamiel is immune to the doctor's attempts to control her now that she has seen the epistemological bankruptcy of language and the possibilities of performance. The originality of *Lamiel* lies in associating the benefits of feminine hypocrisy not with virtue or charm, but with the act of coughing up blood. By placing the blood-soaked sponge in Lamiel's mouth, and coughing up the blood on cue, the *fausse phtisie* scene creates a symptom that previously did not exist. Rather than becoming a passive tuberculosis sufferer, the eponymous heroine *performs* that role. This performance allows Lamiel to remain an active participant in the scene, as the emphasis given to her consent and mocking of Sansfin demonstrate. My argument thus contributes to the work of scholars who have read *Lamiel* as a proto-feminist novel, adding to these analyses that the doctor–patient encounter contains within itself the destruction of a figure of authority through weaponized iconography, and thus the upending of quasi-paternal medical authority itself.

Triangulating the Doctor–Patient Relationship

The question of performance also poses questions about a non-binary doctor–patient relationship in *Lamiel*: the conventionally binary medical relationship would assume that the patient performs for their doctor but, in *Lamiel*, we see that the haemoptysis performance is largely aimed at the Duchesse. Indeed, Sansfin's interest Lamiel is not primarily due to his professional dedication to his patient, but rather due to the fact that he believes that he can influence the Duchesse through his medical relationship with Lamiel. In a plan from March 1842, Stendhal writes that the Doctor wishes to 'saisir la place de remède à l'ennui qui fait le supplice de la duchesse. Cette place est restée vacante depuis la maladie de Lamiel. Après cette première victoire, la vanité de Sansfin prend les ailes, il songe à la fois prendre le P[ucelage] de Lamiel et à se faire épouser par la duchesse' ['to take the place of the remedy for boredom that torments the Duchesse, a position which has remained vacant since Lamiel's illness. After this first victory, Sansfin's vanity spreads its wings; he thinks of both taking Lamiel's virginity and of getting married to the Duchess'].[123] However, despite Sansfin's efforts to execute this triangulation, which is to say his attempt to shift the doctor's focus in the doctor–patient encounter from Lamiel to the Duchesse, the singularity of Lamiel's abject performance of tuberculosis cements her centrality to the novel.

[122] Ibid., III, p. 1014.
[123] Ibid., III, p. 1089.

Nevertheless, *Lamiel* operates in parallel with other novels, suggesting a form of extratextual triangulation. In his analysis of Stendhal's works, Genette proposes 'Un réseau d'interférences' ['A network of overlapping'] between key characters such as between Julien, Fabrice, and Lucien and between Mathilde, Madame de Rênal, Gina Del Dongo, Clélia Conti, and Bathilde de Chasteller. He also highlights a network of paternal antiheroes such as the malevolent doctors Du Poirier and Sansfin, thus suggesting a parallel between *Lucien Leuwen* and *Lamiel*.[124] Given this paradigmatic reading of Stendhal, it is important to note parallel scenes, as well as characters, between the novels. The *faux accouchement* scene of *Lucien Leuwen* briefly mentioned previously in which Bathilde's childbirth is faked, and the *fausse phtisie* scene of *Lamiel*, in which haemoptysis is performed, both produce symptoms out of thin air.[125] Moreover, both scenes restructured and reconfigure the doctor–patient relationship through these remarkable bedside encounters.

Lucien Leuwen focuses on the story of the eponymous hero's career in Nancy and Paris. Lucien falls in love with Bathilde de Chasteller, a young widow, but their blossoming relationship is thwarted by the scheming of Doctor Du Poirier, who co-ordinates a *faux accouchement* in order to make Lucien believe that his beloved has given birth to another man's child. The portrayal of the doctor–patient relationship in *Lucien Leuwen* questions conventional emphasis on the dichotomous nature of doctor and patient. The *faux accouchement* scene falls at the end of the first half of *Lucien Leuwen* and represents the culmination of Du Poirer's attempt to force Lucien from Nancy. Realizing that the eponymous hero has fallen in love with the widow, Bathilde de Chasteller, Du Poirer choreographs a remarkable scene to trick Lucien into thinking that Bathilde has been unfaithful to him. I now quote this passage in full:

> Voici ce qui arriva: à huit heures et demie, dans un moment où Mademoiselle Bérard parlait à la vieille portière, Anne-Marie fit passer dans la cour Leuwen qui, deux minutes après, fut placé dans un retranchement en bois peint qui occupait la moitié de l'antichambre de Madame de Chasteller. De là Leuwen voyait fort bien ce qui se passait dans la pièce voisine et entendait presque tout ce qui se disait dans l'appartement entier.
>
> Tout à coup, il entendit les vagissements d'un enfant à peine né. Il vit arriver dans l'antichambre le docteur essouflé portant l'enfant dans un linge qui lui parut taché de sang.[126]

[124] Ibid., p. 179.

[125] In *La Vie et la Mort de Mina de Vanghel*, Mina attempts to fake a skin disease for which she consults Madame Cramer's doctors. The performativity of Mina's ruse will be discussed in greater detail, but I have excluded this attempt to fake a disease from the present discussion since Mina's plot is independently conceived and executed, and subsequently used to 'trick' a doctor, whereas the *faux accouchement* and *fausse phtisie* scenes involve both doctor and patient throughout.

[126] *ORC*, II, p. 354.

> Here is what happened: at half past eight, while Mademoiselle Bérard was talking to the old porter, Anne-Marie made Leuwen pass into the forecourt and, two minutes later, he found himself placed in a painted wooden side room which occupied half of Madame de Chasteller's antechamber. From there, Leuwen could clearly see what was going on in the adjoining room and could hear nearly everything that was being said in the entire apartment.
>
> Suddenly, he heard the cries of a newborn baby. He saw the breathless doctor arrive in the antechamber, holding the baby in a cloth that seemed to Leuwen to be stained with blood.

To ensure that Lucien correctly interprets what he has just seen, the doctor says to the maid, after commenting on Lucien's prolonged absence from Bathilde's house, that 'Après tout, peut-être l'enfant n'est pas de lui' ['After all, perhaps the child is not his'].[127] The *faux accouchement* scene has generally been dismissed as far-fetched by scholars. For example, although Sandy Petrey demonstrates how the scene exemplifies the duplicitous nature of Orleanist politics, he also admits that 'It would be hard to think of a less credible, more fantastic scene in a realist novel'.[128] However, the scene reveals not only the political context of the novel, but also the non-binary nature of the Stendhalian doctor–patient relationship.

Some pages earlier, in the first instance of what will become a physically abusive doctor–patient relationship, Du Poirier confines Bathilde to her quarters as part of his ploy to force Lucien to flee from Nancy. He tells her friends, 'sous le sceau du secret' ['under the veil of secrecy'] that Bathilde is more ill than first thought, and that 'sa maladie serait longue tout au moins' ['her illness would be long at least'].[129] In an escalation of the violence against Bathilde's body, he deliberately debilitates his patient by cutting her leg, 'Il engagea Madame de Chasteller à souffrir un vésicatoire à la jambe et l'empêcha ainsi de marcher pendant un mois' ['He forced Madame de Chasteller to endure a vesicatory on her leg and thus prevented her from walking for a month'].[130] In order to terrorize her further, and thus place her more firmly under his control, Du Poirier checks her vital signs and carries out the last rites: 'il arriva chez elle d'un air sérieux qui devint sombre en lui tâtant le pouls, et il l'engagea à toutes les cérémonies religieuses qui, en province, sont comprises dans ce seul mot: se faire administrer' ['he arrived in her quarters looking serious and became sombre whilst taking her pulse, and he encouraged her to take all the religious ceremonies which, in the provinces, are understood through this sole word: to be administered'].[131] Du Poirier's efforts to separate Lucien from

[127] *ORC*, II, p. 355.
[128] Sandy Petrey, *In the Court of the Pear King: French Culture and the Rise of Realism* (Ithaca, NY: Cornell University Press, 2005), p. 140.
[129] *ORC*, II, p. 349.
[130] Ibid., II, pp. 349–50.
[131] Ibid., II, p. 353.

Bathilde reach their crescendo in the *faux accouchement* scene, as soon as the doctor discovers that Bathilde's fever has begun to abate. Bathilde is notable as the absent centre of this scene since it is focalized through Lucien, witness to Du Poirier's dramatic production of the bloodied newborn infant, who is secreted in the antechamber of Bathilde's room. Bathilde is thus only evoked *in absentia*. Lucien imagines he is speaking to Bathilde as he says: 'ma chère Bathilde, je ne puis donc plus t'aimer?' ['my dear Bathilde, can I no longer love you?'].[132] Bathilde's absence from *Lucien Leuwen*, forced by Du Poirier, leads Scott to exclude her from her discussion of Stendhal's 'self-inventing heroines' that includes both Mina and Lamiel.[133] Bathilde lacks what Scott terms as the 'joyful egoism' that Lamiel exploits in order to place herself at the heart of the doctor–patient encounter.[134]

By contrast, Beauvoir argues that Bathilde is amongst Stendhal's freedom-loving heroines by foregrounding the negated quality of her freedom. Regarding Bathilde, she writes that her indifference becomes a source of freedom: 'c'est son détachement à l'égard de tout ce qui est secondaire; soumise aux volontés de son père et même à ses opinions, elle n'en conteste pas moins les valeurs bourgeoises par cette indifférence qu'on lui reproche comme un enfantillage et qui est la source de sa gaieté insouciante' ['it her detachment from all that is secondary; submissive to her father's wishes and even to his opinions, she nonetheless challenges bourgeois values through this indifference for which she is criticized as childish and which is the source of her carefree gaiety'].[135] The *faux accouchement* scene exemplifies Beauvoir's argument: although Bathilde is entirely effaced in the scene by Du Poirier and the attention he pays to Lucien, a few pages prior the reader is momentarily privy to her inner thoughts. Whilst doubting that her fever is extraordinary, a hunch that is later proved correct, Bathilde ruminates on the meaning of death: 'Mourir n'est donc que cela! [...] La mort ne serait rien absolument si j'avais M. Leuwen. [...] Au fait, sans lui la vie aurait eu peu de charmes pour moi' ['Dying is only that! [...] Death would be absolutely nothing if I had M. Leuwen. [...] Indeed, without him, life would have had little charm for me'].[136] Bathilde even begins to embrace death and, as such, her narrative 'death', her absence from the *faux accouchement* scene and the rest of the novel, is tantamount to the fulfilment of her desire for release from life.[137] Bathilde is not effaced from *Lucien Leuwen* purely because of Du Poirier's desire to do so, but also because of the structure of the doctor–patient encounter during the *faux accouchement* scene. Thus far the Stendhalian doctor–patient relationship has been understood as binary, principally occupied by the two central actors (*malade* and *médecin*) and defined as

[132] *ORC*, II, p. 356.
[133] Scott, *Stendhal's Less-Loved Heroines*, p. 7.
[134] Ibid., p. 7.
[135] Beauvoir, *Le Deuxième Sexe*, I, p. 380.
[136] *ORC*, II, p. 350.
[137] Ibid., II, p. 350.

an interpersonal dynamic between them. Yet in the *faux accouchement* scene, the patient is almost entirely eliminated; instead, Du Poirier exploits Bathilde's body in order to manipulate Lucien. The *faux accouchement* scene therefore represents both a singular encounter between doctor and patient, albeit with that patient being absent from the narrative, as well as Du Poirer's attempt to triangulate the doctor–patient relationship by aiming the dramatic performance at Lucien. With the presence of three actors—doctor, patient (Bathilde), and target (Lucien)—the doctor–patient relationship is triangulated and made multiple. This triangulated medical relationship notably features two male actors encircling a female patient, but the imagining of an alternative form of the doctor–patient relationship lays the groundwork for its further subversion as we will see in Chapters Three and Four.

Conclusion

Although Sansfin may believe himself to be in control of the bird's execution, and by default Lamiel herself, the recurrence of the execution motif points towards his doomed quasi-paternalistic power. *Lamiel* thus targets the dead bird iconography on which images such as *La Pleureuse* rely, and in which Diderot's 1765 review is intently interested, in order to reveal and resist the quasi-incestuous discourse surrounding young girls. The bird's summary execution recalls the destruction of tyrannical quasi-paternal and incestual power in other Stendhal novels, revealing Lamiel's refusal of these models of power. Furthermore, Lamiel's performance of haemoptysis in the *fausse phtisie* scene extends this subversion further, rendering female patienthood not just active but also abject and performative. It is thus clear that *Lamiel* revolves around a complex interplay between literary and medical discourses, building on Laënnec's symptomology of the disease yet focusing on how the disease is manipulated. At the same time, the novel subverts Romantic conceptions of tuberculosis. We have also seen how *Lucien Leuwen*, and *Lamiel* to a lesser extent, undermine the conventionally binary doctor–patient relationship by triangulating the medical encounter through the introduction of a third party and setting up parallel readings between Stendhal texts.

Understanding Lamiel as an active performer of illness, rather than a passive sufferer, also allows us to reconsider the status of the January 1840 version of the novel in which the *fausse phtisie* scene appears. Schor famously characterizes the later version of the manuscript as representing the 'unwriting' of *Lamiel* and its rebellious heroine, arguing that this version portrays a tamed heroine and is, itself, a more constrained text.[138] In short, the eponymous heroine of *Lamiel* represents a radical model of feminine patienthood thanks to a singular bedside encounter in which the hierarchical and binary nature of the doctor–patient relationship

[138] Schor, *Breaking the Chain*, p. 141.

is uprooted and subverted. Lamiel is thus relatively unique in Stendhal's œuvre, as the narrator of the novel observes: 'Avec son air doux et gai, elle est l'audace même; elle a le courage, plus humain que féminin, de braver votre mépris, et c'est pourquoi elle est inimitable. Regardez-la bien, messieurs, [...] jamais vous n'en verrez une semblable' ['With her gentle and cheerful demeanour, she is daring itself; she is brave enough, more human than feminine, to defy your contempt, and that is why she is inimitable. Take a good look at her, gentlemen, [...] you will never see another like her'].[139]

[139] *ORC*, III, p. 200.

Chapter Three
Medical Narratives and Diseased Bodies: Troubling Encounters in Sand and Balzac

Introduction

Published in 1833, George Sand's elliptical novel *Lélia* revolves around the eponymous heroine who finds herself caught between three potential suitors: the poet Sténio, a former adventurer Trenmor, and a hermit, Magnus. Seeking to reject their advances, Lélia eventually withdraws to a convent where she is found by Sténio. As such, the novel is often read as a story of Lélia's refusal of heteronormative and reproductive sexual relations (an idea to which I will return later), but in this chapter I interpret the text as a narrative that revolves around disease. At the beginning of the novel, Lélia contracts cholera and almost dies, creating the occasion for a dramatic bedside scene. Unlike in *Lamiel*, discussed in Chapter Two, the heroine's affliction is all too real and life-threatening yet like Stendhal's novel, *Lélia* is a biting satire of medicine in the 1830s. The novel was published only one year after the 1832 cholera pandemic which infected one in nineteen Parisians and killed 18,000 people according to reports made in the years after the outbreak.[1] In her autobiographical work *Histoire de ma vie*, Sand recounts how the composition of the novel was determined by contemporary events, including the outbreak of cholera in Paris:

> La République rêvée en juillet aboutissait aux massacres [...]. Le choléra venait de décimer le monde. Le saint-simonisme [...] était frappé de persécution et avortait [...]. L'art aussi avait souillé, par des aberrations déplorables, le berceau de sa réforme romantique. [...] C'est sous le coup de cet abattement profond que j'écrivis *Lélia*.[2]
>
> The Republic dreamed of in July ended in massacres [...]. Cholera had decimated the world. Saint-Simonism [...] was stricken with persecution and had absconded

[1] *Rapport sur les épidémies cholériques de 1832 et 1849 dans les établissements dependant de l'administration générale de l'assistance publique de la ville de Paris* (Paris: Paul Dupont, 1850), p. 152.

[2] George Sand, *Histoire de ma vie*, ed. by Martine Reid (Paris: Gallimard, 2004), pp. 1272–3. Cholera is also repeatedly mentioned by Balzac and Sand in their correspondence to one another during the epidemic's peaks in April and July 1832. See Honoré de Balzac, *Correspondance*, ed. by Roger Pierrot and Hervé Yon, 3 vols (Paris: Gallimard, 2006), I, pp. 501–41.

The Doctor–Patient Relationship and the Nineteenth-Century French Novel. Sarah Jones, Oxford University Press.
© Sarah Jones (2025). DOI: 10.1093/oso/9780198893790.003.0004

> [...]. Art had sullied, by deplorable aberrations, the cradle of its Romantic reform. [...] It was under the influence of this deep dejection that I wrote *Lélia.*

Despite this striking connection between the composition of *Lélia* and the occurrence of the 1832 cholera pandemic, Pierre Reboul dismisses Sand's depiction of cholera as inaccurate and based on her contraction of a less deadly disease in the spring of 1832: 'Mais on doute que Lélia pût sourire, fût-ce de dédain! Ajoutons que Sand n'avait pas été atteinte du choléra, mais, au plus, de la *cholérine*, forme bénigne ou maladie étrangère' ['But it is doubtful that Lélia could smile, even if it were from disdain! Let us add that Sand never had cholera, but, at most, *cholerine*, a benign form or a foreign disease'].[3]

I contest Reboul's statement on two points: firstly, Lélia's alluring smile is surely suggestive of a symbolic meaning since it is simultaneously sardonic and knowing as well as tragically pained. As I will demonstrate in more detail, Lélia's smile embodies her denouncing of medical authority and, on the plane of narration, rejects realistic mimesis that was associated with the doctor's medical gaze. Secondly, Sand's brief illness during the spring of 1832 is significant whether she suffered from cholera or not, since her endurance of similar symptoms must have been a harrowing experience given how the threat of a dehumanizing and anonymous death was all-pervasive in 1832. In a letter to her mother that spring, Sand writes that she had a touch of cholera that was healed with at-home remedies: 'J'ai eu quelque symptômes du choléra, mais si légers qu'une tasse de thé et des couvertures les ont dissipés et que j'ai dormi comme un sonneur jusqu'à midi' ['I had a few cholera symptoms, but so mildly that a cup of a tea and some blankets cleared them and I slept like a slept like a log until midday'].[4] All the same, Sand also insists that 'J'ai été très malade cette nuit, ma chère Maman, à tel point que mes amis et mes portiers ont décidé que j'avais le choléra' ['I was very ill that night, my dear Mother, to such an extent that my friends and porters decided I had cholera'], revealing that, although Sand knew that she had escaped the full force of cholera, she also recognized the potential gravity of her situation.

This chapter argues that Sand's *Lélia* uses cholera and its metaphors to criticize the patriarchal and binary doctor–patient relationship. The bedside scene in *Lélia* appropriates and satirizes contemporary discourse formulated by medical professionals in their vain attempts to understand and treat cholera. Sand finds cholera to be a rich metaphorical nexus of physical symptoms that helps construct an aesthetics of the female body impenetrable to the male doctor's *regard médical.* The novel uses these medical metaphors and discourses to respond to a vision of medicine and its relationship with the female body that is specifically

3 George Sand, *Lélia*, ed. by Pierre Reboul (Paris: Gallimard, 2003), p. 61, n. 1.
4 Ibid., p. 62, n. 2.

Balzacian. I demonstrate Sand's incorporation of the medical discourse of cholera into *Lélia* through, firstly, a satire of the medical inertia around the disease and, secondly, the corporeal metaphors associated with the disease. Comparing *Lélia* to Balzac's *La Peau de chagrin*, of which Sand was an early reader and fervent admirer, and *L'Interdiction*, I demonstrate the extent to which *Lélia* can be read as a rejection of Balzac's realist mode in favour of an idealistic conception of female patienthood. In the final section, however, I question the extent to which Balzac's portrayal of Bianchon as the medical and narratorial lynchpin of *La Comédie humaine* can be believed. In this way, this chapter qualifies the idealistic paternal doctor–patient relationship that the country doctor trope affords Balzac in *Le Médecin de campagne* that I explore in Chapter One. Instead, medicine in Balzac is best understood as deeply ambivalent, oscillating between satire and idealism, and between failure and redemption.

Medical Epistemologies at the Bedside

Isabelle Hoog Naginski describes how the bedside scene in *Lélia* is a 'confrontation of four ideologies' between Trenmor, Doctor Kreyssneifetter, the priest Magnus, and the poet Sténio.[5] As scholars in the critical medical humanities remind us, the patient's bedside is never merely a site for diagnosis and treatment. In this section I contend, however, that in addition to these four ideologies represented by the four men surrounding Lélia's bedside, in a manner reminiscent of *La Peau de chagrin* which will I discuss, Doctor Kreyssneifetter is a singular embodiment of medical inertia in response to the cholera epidemic. Given the backdrop of the 1832 cholera epidemic, Lélia's bedside becomes a battleground between different medical epistemologies and the eponymous heroine's struggle for control over her illness narrative.

Cholera was the most terrifying infectious disease of the nineteenth century, as well as one of the deadliest. It subsumed, and came to define, all that it encountered, as the contemporary Eugène Roch observed in the *Journal des débats* after the first cholera epidemic of 1832: 'Le choléra était tout' ['Cholera was everything'].[6] Despite the ubiquity of cholera according to contemporary observers, scholarship has generally deemed that literary fiction neglected the epidemic. Sontag observes that depictions of cholera were less widespread than diseases such as tuberculosis. She suggests that cholera epidemics, and in particular their propensity to strike the poor and working class, minimize the individualizing effect of other diseases such as tuberculosis.[7] Moïse Le Yaounac has similarly argued that,

[5] Isabelle Hoog Naginski, *George Sand: Writing for Her Life* (New Brunswick, NJ: Rutgers University Press, 1991), p. 123.

[6] Eugène Roch, 'Paris malade; esquisses du jour', *Journal des débats*, 29 September 1832, p. 3.

[7] Susan Sontag, *Illness as Metaphor; and, AIDS and Its Metaphors*, (London: Penguin, 1991), p. 38.

for writers such as Balzac, the reality of epidemics, such as cholera and dysentery, were too horrific to be written.[8] In this section I demonstrate how Sand uses cholera to reveal the divisions within medicine that undermined the doctor's authority over his patient.

The appearance of cholera in Western Europe in the 1830s provoked a profound crisis in medicine. Doctors and scientists both found the disease mystifying, with the result that this crisis undermined the doctor's medical authority within the doctor–patient relationship, and, in some instances, Parisians violently turned against medical professionals.[9] In his classic study of the 1832 cholera pandemic, François Delaporte highlights that one of the major causes of anxiety about contemporary medicine's ability to combat disease lay in the fact that doctors were highly divided in terms of both the causes, and effects, and therefore also the potential treatments for cholera. Theories of cholera's aetiology ranged from hydraulic, to electrical, geological, zoological, and ideas about the disease's pathological effects included suggestions based on Bichat's inflammation model, Magendie's experimental methods, Pinel's theory of nerves, and humoral medicine.[10] Another debate centred on whether cholera spread through miasma or contagion.[11] Because of the proliferation of theories as to cholera's cause, progression, spread, and cure, the medical profession found itself powerless when faced with such a deadly enigma:

> De l'exposition succincte que nous venons de présenter sur la mortalité dans le XIe arrondissement pendant l'invasion du choléra-morbus, nous sommes arrivé [sic] à proclamer cette triste vérité, que beaucoup de médecins se sont trop hâtés de se prononcer dans une maladie sur laquelle, il faut l'avouer, nous n'avons pu encore acquérir que ses données superficielles. Où réside la cause du choléra-morbus? Est-ce dans l'air, dans les émanations terrestres, dans les influences atmosphériques? Qui pourrait l'indiquer? Comment cette cause agit-elle? Est-ce en surexcitant les organes intérieurs des cavités splanchniques? Est-ce en altérant le sang? Qui pourrait résoudre cette dernière question, d'une manière satisfaisante et positive?[12]

[8] Moïse Le Yaouanc, *Nosographie de l'humanité balzacienne* (Paris: Librairie Maloinc, 1959), pp. 273–5. Alexandre Mikhalevitch also finds few references to cholera in his study of Horace Bianchon: 'l'effet d'une probable terreur éprouvée par l'auteur [...] par la manifestation de la fureur des pauvres à l'égard des élites' ['the effect of a probable terror felt by the author [...] by the expression of the poor's anger towards the social elite']. Alexandre Mikhalevitch, *Balzac et Bianchon* (Paris: Honoré Champion, 2014), p. 298.

[9] François Delaporte, *Disease and Civilization: The Cholera in Paris, 1832*, trans. by Arthur Goldhammer (Cambridge, MA; London: MIT Press, 1986), p. 10.

[10] Ibid., pp. 87–9, 93–5, 119–29.

[11] Ibid., pp. 135–9.

[12] Charles-François Tacheron, *Statistique médicale de la mortalité du choléra-morbus dans le XIe arrondissement de Paris pendant les mois d'avril, mai, juin, juillet et août 1832* (Paris: Bechet Jeune, 1832), p. 51.

> From the brief exposition that we have just presented on the death rate in the eleventh arrondissement during the cholera outbreak, we have reached the point of claiming this sad truth, which many doctors have been too hasty to decide on an illness about which, we must admit, we have only superficial data. Where is cholera's cause? Is it in the air, in terrestrial emissions, in atmospheric pressures? What could tell either way? How does this cause work? Is it by overexciting the internal organs of the stomach? By altering the blood? Who could resolve this last question in an affirmative and satisfactory way?

In this passage, Doctor Tacheron condemns doctors for proclaiming to understand cholera when, in fact, they only knew of its most superficial aspects. He lists the fundamental but unanswered questions regarding cholera, asking for an enlightened individual to answer them. The multiplicity of treatments pointed to the professional panic about the causes of, and treatments for, cholera. Suggested treatments included bloodletting with leeches, as advocated by Broussais; a special punch developed by Magendie for which the recipe was a follows: 'Camomille, une pinte; alcool, deux onces; sucre, quatre onces; suc d'un citron' ['Camomile tea, one pint; alcohol, two ounces; sugar, four ounces; lemon juice'].[13] Henri Scoutetten also developed a special heating machine in order to artificially warm the bodies of cholera patients in the hope that treating this symptom would save them from the brink of death.[14] Sand herself was treated with homespun versions of these remedies: in *Histoire de ma vie* she recounts being given 'une tasse de thé' as well as being wrapped in blankets.[15]

This diverse range of treatments manifest themselves in *Lélia* through the negligence, malevolence, and ultimate ambivalence of Doctor Kreyssneifetter. Having received news of Lélia's serious illness, Trenmor and Sténio immediately rush to her bedside. They find Lélia in a horrific state: already blue, she seems to be exhibiting all the symptoms of a cholera victim minutes from death. Yet Kreyssneifetter seems baffled and, despite Trenmor's requests for 'le punch du docteur Magendie' ['Doctor Magendie's concoction'], as well as Lélia's suggestion of 'les adoucissants' ['laxatives'], he remains ambivalent as to their effectiveness, offering the thought: 'Essayons les adoucissants, si vous croyez à la vertu des adoucissants' ['Let's try laxatives, if you believe in the efficacy of laxatives'].[16] Instead, Lélia is only inadvertently exposed to a version of Scoutetten's heating machine after her second convulsion: 'Lélia tomba raide et froide sur le parquet. C'était une dernière, une horrible crise. Sténio la pressa contre son cœur en criant de désespoir. Son cœur

[13] François Magendie, *Leçons sur le choléra-morbus* (Paris: Collège de France, 1832), p. 189.
[14] Henri Scoutetten, *Relation historique et médicale de l'épidemie de choléra qui a régné à Berlin en 1831* (Paris: J. Baillère, 1831), p. 189.
[15] Quoted in Sand, *Lélia*, p. 62 n. 2.
[16] Ibid., p. 62.

était brûlant, ses larmes chaudes tombèrent sur le front de Lélia' ['Lélia fell stiff and cold on the floor. It was one final, horrible seizure. Sténio pressed her against his heart, crying out in despair. His heart was aflame, and his warm tears fell on Lélia's forehead'].[17] By contrast, Kreyssneifetter does precious little other than taking Lélia's pulse: 'Le joli docteur Kreyssneifetter tenait familièrement une main de Lélia dans les siennes et, de temps en temps, il interrogeait le mouvement de l'artère' ['The handsome Doctor Kreyssneifetter held Lélia's hand in his in a familiar way and, now and then, he would scrutinize the movement of the artery'].[18] In his editorial notes on *Lélia*, Reboul compares Kreyssneifetter's cholera treatment to contemporary advice. On the one hand, he attributes Lélia's symptoms to theories of both Magendie and Pinel who, according to Delaporte, were in acrimonious disagreement with one another.[19] On the other hand, he finds that Kreyssneifetter's conviction to 'ne me mêler en rien de cette maladie' ['not interfere with this disease'] suggests an adherence to Pinel's theory of cholera's nervous aetiology.[20]

Rather than portraying specific approaches to treating cholera as Reboul suggests, Kreyssneifetter's conflicting medical approach in fact resonates with the lack of certainty in medical circles about the best course of treatment for cholera. His failure to intervene, and indeed his general ambivalence towards both cholera and his patient, is a striking feature of his treatment of Lélia. When Sténio asks 'Mais que conseillerez-vous, selon votre conscience?' ['But what do you advise, according to your conscience?'] the doctor is indignant: 'À ce mot de conscience, le docteur Kreyssneifetter jeta un regard de compassion moqueuse au jeune poète' ['At the word "conscience", Doctor Kreyssneifetter gave the young poet a mockingly compassionate look'] before explaining that 'Ma conscience m'ordonne de ne rien ordonner du tout, et de ne me mêler en rien de cette maladie' ['My conscience commands me to do nothing, and not to interfere with this disease'].[21] Sand's irony is perceptible here through the doctor's repetitious use of *ordonner* and *rien*, drawing attention to the both the vacuousness of his statement in addition to the cruelty of his abdication of professional and ethical responsibility. The doctor's inertia is explained by his reluctance to commit to a single medical system, thus leading him to biological fatalism: 'Je crois peu à l'influence d'un système quelconque [...]; nous naissons tous avec le principe d'une mort plus ou moins prochaine; nos efforts pour retarder le terme ne font souvent que le hâter' ['I do not strongly believe in the influence of any system [...]; we are all born with the principle of a more or less impending death; our efforts to delay its arrival often only hasten it'].[22] Thus, the doctor advises that patients should stoically accept death: 'Le mieux est de n'y

[17] Ibid., p. 70.
[18] Ibid., p. 61.
[19] Ibid, p. 61 n. 1 and p. 70 n. 3; Delaporte, *Disease and Civilization*, pp. 129–30.
[20] Sand, *Lélia*, p. 63 n. 1.
[21] Ibid., pp. 62–3.
[22] Ibid., p. 63.

pas penser et de l'attendre en oubliant qu'il doit venir' ['The best thing to do is to not think about it and to expect it without forgetting that it must come'].[23] Unlike Benassis or Pascal who, as we saw in Chapter One, find some small consolation in the inevitability and universality of death, here Kreyssneifetter's comments seem painfully callous, particularly in the face of such an agonizing death as that of a cholera victim, and therefore draw attention to how the novel satirizes medicine in this regard.

Due to medicine's failure to provide clear answers as to the workings or treatment of cholera, nineteenth-century doctors often turned to moralizing cures. These are the primary target of Sand's satire of medicine in *Lélia*. In 1832, the Société des amis du peuple encouraged the Parisian poor to protect themselves against cholera, stating that there was only one 'véritable préservatif contre le Choléra, à l'usage surtout de la population malaisée de Paris, c'est de ne point craindre le Choléra; c'est de rester en présence de ce nouvel ennemi, ce qu'elle est partout, courageuse et invincible' ['true protective against cholera, especially for use by the difficult portion of the population of Paris, is not to fear cholera at all, to remain in the presence of this new enemy, which is everywhere, fearless and invincible'].[24] This moralizing tone similarly characterizes Doctor Kreyssneifetter's diagnosis of and advice to Lélia:

> Ce n'est rien, disait-il avec un aimable sourire, rien du tout. C'est le choléra, le choléra-morbus, la chose la plus commune du monde dans ce temps-ci, et la maladie la mieux connue. Rassurez-vous, mon bel ange! vous avez le choléra, une maladie qui tue en deux heures ceux qui ont la faiblesse de s'en effrayer, mais qui n'est point dangereuse pour les esprits fermes comme les nôtres. Ne vous effrayez donc pas, aimable étrangère! Nous sommes ici deux qui ne craignons pas le choléra, vous et moi défions le choléra! Faisons peur à ce vilain spectre, à ce hideux monstre qui fait dressser les cheveux au genre humain. Raillons le choléra! c'est la seule manière de le traiter.[25]

> It's nothing, he said with a friendly smile, nothing at all. It's cholera, cholera morbus, the most common thing in the world nowadays and the best-known disease. Rest assured, my beautiful angel, you have cholera, a disease which kills in two hours those who are weak enough to be afraid of it, but which is not dangerous for stoic minds like ours. So don't be afraid, lovely stranger! There are two of us here who are not afraid of cholera, we shall overcome it, you and I! Let's scare this awful phantom, this hideous monster that makes mankind's hair stand on end. Let's laugh at cholera. That's the only way to treat it.

[23] Ibid., p. 63.
[24] Société des amis du peuple, *De la civilisation* (Paris: Carpentier de Méricourt, 1832), p. 4.
[25] Sand, *Lélia*, pp. 61–2.

By asserting that, since cholera was a moral disease, the best cure was the cultivation of moral fortitude and the rejection of fear, *Lélia* thus ironizes the medical profession's contemporary confusion about the causes and treatments for cholera. Sand's use of the third person plural is an ironic take on the doctor–patient relationship: the doctor believes, or at least be trying to make the patient believe, that they are fighting a joint enterprise. But this third person plural is disingenuous: the doctor's lack of practical advice only isolates the patient further, and thus Sand's novel uses the medico-historical context of the 1832 cholera epidemic to criticize positivist science by ironizing it through the doctor–patient encounter at Lélia's bedside.

Moreover, *Lélia* uses this satirical doctor–patient encounter to criticize the epistemological structures on which contemporary medical science was built. Lélia rejects scientific observation: given Kreyssneifetter's inertia, Lélia caustically excuses the 'philosophe' ['philosopher'] from her bedside: 'Alors comme il se fait tard, bonsoir! N'interrompez pas plus longtemps votre précieux sommeil' ['So, since it's late, good evening! Do not allow your precious sleep to be interrupted any longer'].[26] However, the doctor defends his presence by demonstrating his personal sacrifice to his profession: 'je suis bien ici, je me plais à suivre les progrès du mal. J'étudie, j'aime mon métier de passion, et je sacrifie volontiers mes plaisirs et mon repos, je sacrifierais ma vie s'il le fallait pour le bien de l'humanité' ['I'm fine here; I like to follow the disease's progress. I study, I love my profession with a passion, and I willingly sacrifice my pleasures and my rest. I would sacrifice my life if I had to for the good of humanity'].[27] The doctor goes on to define his *métier* as follows: 'Je console, j'encourage [...]. Je la constate, je l'observe, j'assiste au dénouement et je profite de mes observations' ['I console, I encourage [...]. I see it, I watch it, I watch the outcome, and I enjoy my observations'].[28] Although Kreyssneifetter makes some gesture towards the empathetic role that a doctor should play, the emphasis here is on his skills as a cold-hearted observer of the ilk evoked by Foucault in *Naissance de la clinique*, one who takes a sadistic pleasure in his observations of the painful progression of disease.

The novel's rejection of medical observation, and the underpinning Enlightenment values of objectivity and universalism, are underscored by the novel's most famous maxim: '*Savoir*, ce n'est pas *pouvoir*' ['Knowing is not power'].[29] Naginski compares this phrase to the famous line from *La Peau de chagrin*: 'Voir, n'est-ce pas savoir?' ['Seeing, isn't that knowing?'].[30] In that novel the *antiquaire* recounts a desire for visual mastery equated with materialized knowledge: 'Ma seule ambition a été de voir. Voir, n'est-ce pas savoir? [...] Que reste-t-il d'une

[26] Ibid., p. 63.
[27] Ibid., p. 63.
[28] Ibid., p. 63.
[29] Ibid., p. 120.
[30] Naginski, *George Sand*, p. 133.

possession matérielle? Une idée' ['My only ambition was to see. Seeing, isn't that knowing? [...] What remains from a material possession? An idea'].[31] Not only does *Lélia* question this analogy between *savoir* and *pouvoir*, as Naginski argues, but Sand's novel demonstrates the inefficacy of medicine when it is seen from the patient's perspective. Lélia asks Kreyssneifetter 'vous ne croyez donc pas à la médicine?' ['you don't believe in medicine?'], to which the doctor evasively replies that 'l'étude de l'anatomie et la connaissance du corps humain avec ses altérations et ses infirmités, c'est là une science positive' ['the study of anatomy and the knowledge of the human body with its alterations and infirmities, that is a positivist science'].[32] What good does the study of the body do if Kreyssneifetter's response to Lélia's cholera is to advise her to be indignant, rather than to heal her physically or emotionally? Exasperated, Lélia declares that science has deserted the doctor and therefore her: 'je vois que le médecin m'abandonne. [...] Quand je sentirai le courage m'abandonner, je le ferai appeler, afin qu'il me donne des conseils de stoïcisme et que je meure en riant de l'homme et de sa science' ['I can see that the doctor has given up on me. [...] When I feel courage leaving me, I will call him, so that he can me give me his stoic advice and so that I can die laughing at this man and his science'].[33] The doctor–patient encounter in *Lélia* thus questions the efficacy and supposedly inherent utility of the medical gaze within the medical relationship. I return to the question of the medical gaze and its (failed) penetration of the diseased female body in the following section of this chapter.

The satire of medical discourse in *Lélia* is not just a response to the medical profession's failures during the 1832 cholera pandemic, but also represents a riposte to a conception of medical authority that characterizes Balzac's *La Comédie humaine*. *Lélia* therefore challenges not just the medical establishment itself, but a specific literary discourse of and about medicine. In Chapter One, *Le Médecin de campagne* emerged as a novel that relies on an idealized conception of medicine, one which turns back the clock on the 1789 Revolution and uses the doctor–patient relationship to heal the doctor's adopted community. Sand was famously an early reader and admirer of Balzac's *La Peau de chagrin*, published merely three years before *Lélia*. There is critical precedence of comparing these two novels: Manon Mathias uses Balzac's novel to establish ideas of visual instability and fluidity on which Sand's later novel build.[34] As will be discussed in further detail, Nigel Harkness uses *La Peau de chagrin* as a 'paradigmatic text for thinking desire' against which he compares Sand's *Lélia*.[35] Although Balzac may satirize three of Raphaël's

[31] Honoré de Balzac, *La Peau de chagrin*, ed. by Nadine Satiat (Paris: Flammarion, 1996), p. 89; Manon Mathias, *Vision in the Novels of George Sand* (Oxford: Oxford University Press, 2016), p. 31.
[32] Sand, *Lélia*, p. 64.
[33] Ibid., p. 64.
[34] Mathias, *Vision in the Novels of George Sand*, pp. 21–3.
[35] Nigel Harkness, *Men of Their Words: The Poetics of Masculinity in George Sand's Fiction* (London: Legenda, 2007), p. 121.

doctors as pretentious and garrulous, I demonstrate, firstly, that Horace Bianchon emerges as a both a moral anchor for the scene and thus medicine's saving grace and, secondly, that *Lélia* responds to this portrayal of the medical relationship. Whereas *Lélia* depicts a singular doctor–patient relationship observed by other bedside attendees; the scene from *La Peau de chagrin* oscillates around a bedside encounter in which the patient has a simultaneous encounter with four different doctors, thus rendering plural the usually binary doctor–patient relationship.

La Peau de chagrin is profoundly concerned with what Balzac saw as the widespread disillusionment of post-1789 France. In the dinner-party scene at the end of the novel's first part we read that 'la liberté enfante l'anarchie, l'anarchie conduit au despotisme, et le despotisme ramène à la liberté' ['freedom gives birth to anarchy, anarchy leads to despotism, and despotism leads back to freedom'], which is 'le cercle vicieux dans lequel tournera toujours le monde moral' ['the vicious cycle that the moral world always turns in'].[36] The oscillation of despotism and freedom between their opposite positions of laws and morals means that the consequent power vacuum has now been filled by speculation. A banker sardonically cries out 'Buvons donc à l'imbécillité du pouvoir qui nous donne tant de pouvoir sur les imbéciles!' ['So let's drink to the stupidity of power that give us so much power over fools!'][37] Here I argue that this disillusionment with political life extends to a disenchantment with both medical epistemology and medical practice that is articulated through an iconic bedside encounter during which different medical ideologies encounter one another and a patient.

Having become critically ill by dint of his use of the magical donkey skin to fulfil his desires, Raphaël wakes one morning to find himself surrounded by four doctors who prod and poke him whilst submitting him to heavy-handed medical examinations. The reader is immediately alerted to the fact that three of these four doctors are representatives of the competing contemporary medical doctrines of Analysis, Vitalism, and Eclecticism: 'les trois systèmes entres lesquels flottent les connaissances humaines étaient là devant lui' ['before him were the three systems between which knowledge about the human body flits'].[38] Rather than representing the great and good of contemporary medicine, these doctors embody the stasis of early nineteenth-century medicine. The first doctor, Doctor Brisset, is the representative of the Analysis school. Brisset is designated the modern successor of Cabanis and of Bichat who together 'voient en l'homme un être fini, uniquement sujet aux lois de sa propre organisation, et dont l'état normal ou les anomalies délétères s'expliquent par des causes évidentes' ['see in man a finite being, uniquely subject to the laws of his own organization, and of which the normal state or the harmful anomalies are explained by obvious causes'].[39] Cabanis and Bichat

[36] Balzac, *La Peau de chagrin*, pp. 105–6.
[37] Ibid., p. 106.
[38] Ibid., p. 284.
[39] Ibid., p. 285.

were empiricists primarily occupied with analysing and understanding tissue: as Erwin H. Ackerknecht states, the 'medicine of observation' favoured in the nineteenth century was 'fathered by a philosophy of observation' of which doctors like Cabanis and Bichat were the primary proponents.[40] The second doctor to be introduced to Raphaël is Doctor Caméristus. Caméristus represents the Vitalist school, the theory that life depends on a singular vital force, since he 'voyait dans la vie humaine un principe élevé, secret, un phénomène inexplicable qui se joue des bistouris, trompe la chirurgie, échappe aux médicaments de la pharmaceutique, aux *x* de l'algèbre, aux démonstrations de l'anatomie' ['sees in human life a secret, elevated principle, an inexplicable phenomenon that toys with scalpels, deceives surgery, escapes drugs, the x of algebra, and dissections'].[41] The founding premise of *La Peau de chagrin*, the idea that the magic skin grants wishes only by draining Raphaël of his life force is consistent with the vitalist doctrine of a single, universal, life-giving fluid to which Balzac roughly adhered: 'la volonté humaine était une force matérielle semblable à la vapeur' ['human will was a material force similar to steam'].[42] However, Caméristus's Vitalist convictions render him an ineffectual doctor who scorns all forms of medical intervention: '[il] se rit [des] efforts [d'autres médecins]' ['he laughed at the efforts of other doctors'] since he maintains that life is ultimately governed by 'une espèce de flamme intangible, invisible, soumis à quelque loi divine, et qui reste souvent au milieu d'un corps condamné par nos arrêts, comme elle déserte aussi les organisations les plus viables' ['a type of intangible, invisible flame, subject to some divine law, and which often remains in the midst of a body otherwise condemned by our own judgements, as it also deserts the most viable organisms'].[43]

Finally, Doctor Maugredie, the doctor of the Eclectic school, could be interpreted as a literary incarnation of François Magendie through a manipulation of the latter's surname to form an onomastic pun (Magendie/Maugredie). Magendie was famed for his heavy use of live vivisection and, in *La Peau de chagrin* Maugredie is described as a Rabelaisian 'Panurge de l'école' ['Panurge of the school'], the 'roi de l'observation' ['king of observing'], and a 'grand explorateur' ['great explorer'].[44] However, he is also a 'grand railleur' ['big teaser'] and, finding good elements in all medical theories, Maugredie refuses to adopt any of them: '[il]

[40] Ackerknecht, *Medicine at the Paris Hospital*, p. 3. Ackerknecht also observes the literary interest in Cabanis's work by observing his spectral presence in the works of authors such as Stendhal, Sainte-Beuve, and Flaubert. See Ackerknecht, *Medicine at the Paris Hospital*, p. 197.

[41] Balzac, *La Peau de chagrin*, pp. 285–6. According to Laurence Brockliss and Colin Jones, vitalists were uninterested in morbid anatomy and instead 'confined the study of disease to the observable' and thus the patient's body. See Brockliss and Jones, *The Medical World of Early Modern France*, p. 436.

[42] Balzac, *La Peau de chagrin*, p. 162. Balzac's interest in a mysterious vital fluid that supported all life forms goes some way to explain his interest in the work of Mesmer and Swedenborg. See Melissa Marcus, *The Representation of Mesmerism in Honoré de Balzac's 'La Comédie humaine'* (New York: Peter Lang, 1995).

[43] Balzac, *La Peau de chagrin*, p. 286.

[44] Ibid., p. 286.

prétendait que le meilleur système médical était de n'en point avoir, et de s'en tenir aux faits' ['he claimed that the best medical system was to not have one, and to stick to the facts'].[45] Maugredie is therefore the 'homme des tentatives désespérées' ['man of desperate attempts']: a man of great ideas and skill but with limited convictions.[46] The inertia of the doctors in attendance at this bedside encounter thus encapsulates Raphaël's sense of disillusionment: he is disappointed by medicine and particularly in his doctors' ability to diagnose effectively or even treat his illness. In *La Peau de chagrin*, then, society and science have been corroded by 'un effroyable sentiment d'égoïsme' ['a dreadful feeling of selfishness'] which is the 'lèpre actuelle' ['current leprosy'] of France after 1789.[47] Nineteenth-century medicine had thus become fragmented and, in *La Peau de chagrin*, the polyphonic doctor–patient encounter demonstrates how this fragmentation to the ordinary hierarchal nature of medicine, which had seen the authoritative doctor preside over the patient, as in *Le Médecin de campagne*.

However, the bedside scene of *La Peau de chagrin* contains one redemptive hope for the medical profession: Bianchon. According to Anne-Marie Lefevre, Bianchon is an 'astre' in the constellation of *La Comédie humaine*.[48] In *La Peau de chagrin*, Bianchon is described as wise and modest, a friend of Rastignac, and with an illustrious career surely ahead of him.[49] Bianchon acts as an arbiter between the doctors of different doctrines: he tries to present a united front to the patient, since professional unanimity allows the doctors to take immediate and decisive action: 'Ces messieurs ont unaniment reconnu la nécessité d'une application immédiate de sangsues' ['These men were unanimous in recognizing the necessity of an immediate application of leeches'].[50] Bianchon is the only doctor able to relate to Raphaël humanely, since he is the only doctor who slowly explains the medical jargon and underpinning epistemology of his colleagues' staunch positions. According to Bianchon, the doctors are 'logiques' ['logical'] since 'Caméristus sent, Brisset examine, Maugredie doute' ['Caméristus feels, Brisset examines, Maugredie doubts'] which mirrors the makeup of man who has 'une âme, un corps et une raison' ['a soul, a body, and a logical mind'].[51] Therefore, there will always be humanity, both in the form of the patient and in the humane doctor, in medicine: 'il y aura toujours de l'homme dans la science humaine' ['there will always be man in human sciences'].[52]

[45] Ibid., p. 286.
[46] Ibid., p. 286.
[47] Ibid., p. 108.
[48] Anne-Marie Lefevre, 'Bianchon, un astre du cosmos balzacien', *L'Année balzacienne*, 16 (1995), 311–50.
[49] Balzac, *La Peau de chagrin*, pp. 284–5.
[50] Ibid., p. 291.
[51] Ibid., p. 292.
[52] Ibid., p. 292.

As we saw in the 'Introduction''s discussion of *Le Père Goriot*, for Bianchon, the aim of medicine is not to accurately diagnose and then heal a patient but to aid the patient's own healing; 'nous ne guérissons pas, nous aidons à guérir' ['we do not heal, we facilitate healing'].[53] Amidst the chaotic bedside consultation, Bianchon is a redemptive figure for medicine and a moral anchor in the scene, asserting the importance of the patient's illness narrative and humanity rather than placing them in the service of science. By placing the patient's physical and moral health above his own financial or political interests, Bianchon is a quintessential *robe noire* whose virtues are expounded in *Le Médecin de campagne*: 'les trois robes noires [sont] le prêtre, l'homme de loi, le médecin; l'un panse les plaies de l'âme, l'autre celles de la bourse, le dernier celles du corps; ils représentent la société dans ses trois principaux termes d'existence: la conscience, le domaine, la santé' ['the three black robes [are] the priest, the lawyer, the doctor: one heals the wounds of the soul, the other those of the family estate, the other the wounds of the body; they represent society in its three principle terms of existence: conscience, estate, and health'].[54] Although the plural doctor–patient encounter in *La Peau de chagrin* illustrates the protagonist's profound disillusionment with nineteenth-century medical epistemology and practice, the moral anchor of a young Bianchon goes some way in redeeming the doctor's authority within the doctor–patient relationship. In this way, for all the novel's disenchantment with medical science, the disappointing bedside encounter between Raphaël and his three warring doctors ends in the idealization of Bianchon as an exceptional and profoundly humane medical practitioner.

In *La Peau de chagrin*, Bianchon is introduced as 'le plus distingué [...] des nouveaux médecins' ['the most distinguished [...] of new doctors'].[55] In *Lélia*, the doctor's youth is exaggerated for the sake of satire. Kreyssneifetter is continuously characterized as young: he is 'le docteur imberbe' ['the beardless doctor'].[56] Bianchon adopts a gentle paternal approach to the care of his patient, questioning not only his colleagues' claim to the patient's illness narrative through their understanding of Raphaël's disease, but reaffirming the patient's sovereignty over his experience. The doctor's exaggeratedly tender age renders his paternalistic bedside manner pompous and patronizing: he speaks in a tone which is 'doucereux et protecteur' ['soft and protective'] to the patient whom he calls 'ma belle enfant' ['my beautiful child'].[57] Unlike Raphaël, a hapless victim of his three in-fighting doctors and whose cause is championed only by Bianchon, Lélia, 'avec un sang-froid

[53] Ibid., p. 292.

[54] Balzac, *Le Médecin de campagne*, passim. Indeed, Bianchon's failure to rigidly adopt a specific doctrine in *La Peau de chagrin* adds further weight to Lefevre's argument that he is a composite of a range of medical figures from the period. See Lefevre, 'Bianchon, un astre du cosmos balzacien'.

[55] Balzac, *La Peau de chagrin*, p. 285.

[56] Sand, *Lélia*, p. 63.

[57] Ibid., pp. 61, 63.

caustique' ['with a caustic coolness'], repels Kreyssneifetter's attempt at patient care.[58] Sand further unpicks the doctor's claim to medical authority by feminizing him in the spirit of a Romantic hero. He is 'le joli docteur' ['the handsome doctor'] and 'un charmant homme tout jeune, blond, vermeil, au sourire nonchalant, à la main blanche' ['a charming young man, blond, rosy-cheeked, with a nonchalant smile and pale, youthful hands'].[59] Lélia appropriates virile masculine power for herself and takes back control of her own narrative. In the only full-length portrait of Lélia, which shows her attending a ball thrown by a famous musician, her appearance evokes the dark garb of the *robes noires*:

> Le manteau de Lélia était moins noir, moins velouté que ses grands yeux couronnés d'un sourcil mobile. La blancheur mate de son visage et de son cou se perdait dans celle de sa vaste fraise et la froide respiration de son sein impénétrable ne soulevait pas même le satin noir de son pourpoint et les triples rangs de sa chaîne d'or.[60]

> Lélia's coat was less black, less velvety than her large eyes that were crowned with expressive eyebrows. The dull whiteness of her face and neck were lost in that of her vast ruff, and the cold breath of her impenetrable chest did not even lift the black satin of her doublet and the triple rows of her gold chain.

In this passage, we see the incorporation of Lélia's impenetrability into the sartorial synecdoche of the male professional. Lélia's adoption of dark masculine clothes signals not only her sexual impenetrability, but equally her appropriation of the clothes used by male professionals to assert their authority.[61] In *La Peau de chagrin*, women are shown to be as impenetrable as professional men: 'Les prêtres, les magistrats et les femmes ne dépouillent jamais leur robe entièrement' ['Priests, magistrates, and women never entirely take off their robes'].[62] Not only does *Lélia* constitute a criticism of Balzac's idealized 'good doctor', but the novel exposes how this idealization is founded on gendered clichés which the radical eponymous heroine defiantly overturns, as the priest Magnus later admits, Lélia's 'puissance est supérieure à la mienne' ['Lélia's strength is superior to mine'].[63] In the third section of this chapter, I demonstrate how, in Sand's parody of Bianchon, the nature of the relationship between medicine, the doctor–patient relationship, and narrative style is at stake.

[58] Ibid., p. 62.
[59] Ibid., p. 61.
[60] Ibid., p. 45.
[61] For the theme of transvestism in Sand, see Jacinta Wright, '"S'habiller du vêtement du maître": George Sand et le travesti intertextuel', in *George Sand: pratiques et imaginaires de l'écriture*, ed. by Brigitte Diaz and Isabelle Hoog Naginski (Caen: Presses universitaires de Caen, 2017), pp. 95–103.
[62] Balzac, *La Peau de chagrin*, pp. 171–2.
[63] Sand, *Lélia*, p. 65.

La Peau de chagrin and *Lélia* both use a doctor–patient encounter at the patient's bedside to satirize modern medicine, and the shared episodic nature of both scenes draws attention to the peripherality of the medical plots to their respective novels. Nevertheless, both scenes are rich in metaphorical meaning. *Lélia* uses a similar scene as *La Peau de chagrin* to satirize medical responses to the cholera epidemic of 1832, thus locating her novel in the historical realities of its inception. Unlike *La Peau de chagrin*, *Lélia* does not provide the reader with a solution to medical inefficacy by including an exceptional, redemptive doctor figure. Instead, the eponymous heroine is forced to seize control over her illness narrative from the polyphony of medical opinion that her doctor represents. *La Peau de chagrin* instead multiplies the bilateral doctor–patient relationship through the presence of the three in-fighting doctors. But, in the case of Balzac, the patient's disillusionment makes way for an idealized 'good doctor' who, through an equally idealized doctor–patient relationship, reaffirms Raphaël's humanity which his doctors otherwise ignore.

Corporeal Struggles

The medical debate in *Lélia* is not, however, an abstract discussion about cholera, but is instead organized around the doctor's lack of knowledge regarding the eponymous heroine's afflicted body. Understanding the interweaving between embodied experience and personal narrative is similarly a key preoccupation for doctors and scholars within the medical humanities: Kirmayer, for example, points out the propensity for the narrated body to fragment into metaphor rather than to form a coherent narrative or plot.[64] The body is also an essential component of the doctor–patient relationship: the doctor's superior medical or scientific understanding of the patient's body may cause a sense of powerlessness or frustration for the patient, particularly given the connection between the body and sense of self.[65] We see this dynamic in *Lélia*: Kreyssneifetter proclaims that nothing is wrong with Lélia physically, challenging her own experience of illness. Yet, because of this response, the text draws attention to the corporeality of its eponymous heroine, focusing attention on ways in which bodies possess their own language that can bespeak of suffering, pain, and other facets of illness that are determined by socio-cultural environments as well as biological and physical factors.[66] In the following section I argue that these corporeal concerns are central to understanding how Sand's *Lélia* uses cholera as a source of metaphors

[64] Kirmayer, 'Broken Narratives', p. 155.

[65] Ezekiel J. Emanuel and Linda L. Emanuel, 'Four Models of the Physician-Patient Relationship', *JAMA: The Journal of the American Medical Association*, 267.16 (1992), p. 11.

[66] For a general discussion of these themes, see *Body Talk in the Medical Humanities: Whose Language?*, ed. by Jennifer Patterson and Francia Kinchington (Newcastle upon Tyne: Cambridge Scholars Publishing, 2019).

that articulate physical impermeability and female resistance. I demonstrate that, whereas *Lélia* is ordinarily read from the perspective of the desiring male gaze, the text also works to rebuff and reject the medical gaze of the doctor.[67] Indeed, the *regard médical* is not entirely distinct from the male gaze, since the male dominance of the male profession in the nineteenth century guaranteed that all medical gazes were surely male. Foucault claims that this gender divide meant that the doctor–patient relationship was erotically charged, referring to 'le vocabulaire faiblement érotisé de la "rencontre" et du "couple médecin–malade"' ['the weakly eroticized vocabulary of the "encounter" between the "doctor–patient couple"'].[68] The metaphors of impenetrable, marmoreal coldness used by Sand, that emanate from the symptoms of cholera itself, reject this projection of the medical desire for knowledge and technological penetration onto the bedside.[69] The doctor–patient encounter is the site at which these features are drawn together, thereby reconfiguring the hierarchical nature of the doctor–patient relationship.

During an attack of cholera, the patient's body became hyper-corporeal in the sense that the disease rendered all the body's normal functions both visible and repulsive. The historian Richard Evans argues that, whereas the 'pale and interesting' look associated with tuberculosis could be co-opted into a Romantic bourgeois sensibility, cholera could not. He instead observes how the symptomology of cholera threatened nineteenth-century bourgeois sensibility:

> The blue, 'corrugated', appearance of the skull and the dull, sunken eyes of sufferers transformed their bodies from those of recognizable people [...] into the living death within a matter of hours. Worse still, the massive loss of bodily fluids, the constant vomiting and defecating of vast quantities of liquid excreta, were horrifying and deeply disgusting in an age which, more than any other, sought to conceal bodily functions from itself. Bourgeois society [...] took increasing pains [...] to make private the grosser physical acts of daily living and to pretend that they did not exist.[70]

In a similar vein, Sontag writes that 'Cholera is the kind of fatality that [...] simplified a complex self, reducing it to a sick environment. The disease that individualizes, that sets a person in relief against the environment, is tuberculosis'.[71] Despite Evans's and Sontag's characterization of cholera as dehumanizing disease

[67] Naginski, *George Sand*, pp. 107–35; Schor, *George Sand and Idealism*, pp. 55–68. Nigel Harkness argues that that *Lélia* presents 'a troubling vision of desire as an uncontrolled, multiform force'; Harkness, *Men of Their Words*, p. 123.

[68] Foucault, *Naissance de la clinique*, p. 12.

[69] Lisa Downing, *Desiring the Dead: Necrophilia and Nineteenth-Century French Literature* (Oxford: Legenda, 2003), p. 11. See also Jacinta Wright, 'Romancing the Dead; Death and Desire in George Sand's *Lélia*', *Irish Journal of French Studies*, 1.1 (2001), 57–66. For an examination of marmoreality more generally, see Peter Cryle, 'Le Marbre féminin', *Revue des sciences humaines*, 271 (2003), 147–55.

[70] Richard J. Evans, *Death in Hamburg: Society and Politics in the Cholera Years, 1830–1910* (New York: Penguin Books, 2005), p. 229.

[71] Sontag, *Illness as Metaphor*, p. 38.

because of the havoc it wreaks on the body, Sand's resistance to medical authority is primarily achieved through a depiction of an impenetrable body, one which resists not just the male medical gaze but also the threat of an environment riddled with contagion and sickness. Naginski draws attention to how 'Lélia, whose blue illness is a metaphor for her despair, is paralyzed by her incapacity to act in the world, to participate in society', suggesting a connection between Lélia's cholera and her feminized *mal du siècle* outlined by Margaret Waller.[72]

Contemporary medical writers of cholera are most often found repeatedly horrified by the effects that cholera would produce on the infected body. Cholera symptoms included the profuse and sudden production of watery diarrhoea, vomiting, and cramps, as well as the blue-tinged skin synonymous with the disease. Excruciating stomach cramps could cause the patient to writhe uncontrollably in pain, and white 'rice-paper' diarrhoea was an unmistakable symptom. Joseph-Claude-Anthelme Récamier described this process as: 'Le malade est pris presque en même temps de vertiges, de vomissements et de diarrhées, avec des crampes douloureuses dans les membres' ['The patient is seized almost simultaneously with dizziness, vomiting, and diarrhoea, and with painful cramps in the limbs'].[73] *Cyanose* or *facies cholérique* were responsible for the blue appearance of the skin that felt cold to the touch, and Doctor Fabre recorded a generalized coldness that affected most of the patient's body: 'Facies cadavérique, teinte violette ou livide de la face et des mains, altération profonde des traits et de la voix, yeux caves secs [...]; refroidissement glacial des membres, du nez, de la face, quelquefois de la langue, haleine froide'[74] ['Cadaver-like features, violet or pallid tint of the face and hands, sunken features and a deepened voice, dry sunken eyes [...]; icy cold are the limbs, nose, forehead, sometimes the tongue, with a cold breath'].

Most harrowing of all was cholera's capacity for *cadavérisation*, turning the patient into a corpse before their death. As Doctor Arrambide wrote: 'La figure est cadavérique et d'un aspect particulier; la peau donne au toucher la sensation de fraîcheur qu'une grenouille produirait à la main; le pouls disparaît entièrement; tout le corps devient froid comme du marbre et d'une couleur plombée ou livide, en commençant par les extrémités' ['The face is cadaverous and of a particular appearance; the skin is cold to the touch, similar to holding a frog; the pulse disappears entirely; the whole body becomes as cold as marble with a leaden or pallid colour beginning in the extremities'].[75] These horrifying effects of cholera was responsible for popular rumours regarding isolated cases of doctors declaring

[72] Naginski, *George Sand*, p. 124; Margaret Waller, *The Male Malady: Fictions of Impotence in the French Romantic Novel* (New Brunswick, NJ: Rutgers University Press, 1993), pp. 136–75.

[73] Joseph-Claude-Anthelme Récamier, *Recherches sur le traitement du choléra morbus* (Paris: Gabon, 1832), pp. 25–6.

[74] Antoine François Hippolyte Fabre, *Du choléra morbus; ou, guide des practiciens dans la connaissance et le traitement de cette maladie* (Paris: Germer Baillière, 1832), p. 8.

[75] J. B. Arrambide, *Explication des symptômes du choléra-morbus, des apparences cadavériques, et de ses méthodes curatives, par des données physiologiques* (Paris: Éverat, 1832), pp. 6–7.

patients' deaths whilst they were still alive: the violinist Niccolò Paganini's doctors pronounced the maestro's due due to his cholera-like symptoms and the disease's ghoulish aping of death. During Paganini's disease, but in the year before the pandemic, they wrote:

> Le système nerveux s'y associe d'une manière si remarquable qu'il se déclare une catalepsie qui le tient tout un jour dans un état de mort apparente. Sa famille désolée croit qu'il a cessé de vivre, et il était déjà enveloppé dans le linceul funéraire et prêt à mettre dans le cercueil, lorsqu'un léger mouvement révéla aux assistans qu'il vivait encore.[76]

> The nervous system becomes involved [in the disease] in such a remarkable way that it develops a catalepsy which keeps the patient in state of apparent death for an entire day. His distressed family believe that he has ceased to live, and he was already wrapped in the burial shroud and was ready to be placed in the coffin, when a slight movement revealed to those present the fact that he was still alive.

Paganini's corpse-like appearance almost results in him being buried alive and, more broadly, interest in taphophobia peaked during the nineteenth century due to cholera's ability to ape death, inspiring images such as the Romantic painter Antoine Wiertz's *L'Inhumation précipitée* in 1854. Cholera, then, was a primordially distressing disease, suddenly striking down ordinary people who would suddenly lose control of their bowels and rapidly giving them a ghoulish blue tinge. The patient's harrowing appearance would quickly give them the appearance of a corpse, foreshadowing their inevitable death.

The fact that Lélia's condition is hyper-physical, insofar as cholera heightened and exposed the body's normal functions, means that her body is rendered visible, albeit unreadable. Through her depiction of the doctor–patient encounter, Sand's novel thus demonstrates the aesthetic potential of the disease to rebel against the paradigms of medical vision and narrative knowledge embedded in the medical relationship. Thompson persuasively demonstrates the corporeal dimension of *Lélia*, particularly regarding gender, writing that *Lélia* 'is a novel which refuses realism and instead rewrites the nineteenth-century model of the easily obtainable feminine body yearned for and ultimately secured by a male hero'.[77] Building on this observation, and bearing in mind Sand's description of her own cholera-like symptoms in a letter to her mother in April 1832, I argue that *Lélia* uses cholera's

[76] Bennati and Miquel, 'Notice physiologique sur Paganini', *Revue de Paris*, 26 (Paris, 1831), pp. 54–5. For this reference I am indebted to Nina Athanassoglou-Kallmyer's excellent article on the death of Paganini. See Nina Athanassoglou-Kallmyer, 'Blemished Physiologies: Delacroix, Paganini, and the Cholera Epidemic of 1832', *The Art Bulletin*, 83.4 (2001), 686–710.

[77] Hannah Thompson, *Taboo: Corporeal Secrets in Nineteenth-Century France*, (Oxford: Legenda, 2013), p. 25.

symptomology as a rich nexus of metaphors to repel the penetrating male gaze away from the female body during the medical encounter. After hearing of Lélia's serious illness and possible death, Trenmore and Sténio rush to her bedside. The abject, undeniably physical reality of cholera is the first thing that strikes them since they find the eponymous heroine 'couchée sur un sofa; ses joues avaient un reflet bleu, ses yeux semblaient s'être retirés sous l'arc profond de ses sourcils. Un grand pli traversait son front, ordinairement si poli et si blanc' ['Lying on a sofa; her cheeks glinted blue, her eyes seemed to have receded beneath the deep arch of her eyebrows. Her forehead, usually so smooth and white, was traversed by a large wrinkle'].[78] Lélia's sunken eyes and blue-tinged skin echo the most widely recognized symptoms of cholera; her creased forehead suggests the agony of the severe stomach cramps caused by the disease. As per contemporary observations of cholera, Lélia's extremities are the most notably discoloured: she talks to Magnus 'en l'attirant vers elle de sa main froide et bleuâtre' ['pulling him towards her with her cold bluish hand'].[79] Lélia's violent convulsions increase her cadaverous appearance: she 'tomba mourante' ['fell dying'] and a few pages later asks 'Suis-je déjà morte?' ['Am I already dead?'].[80] Lélia's thanatological question, has she already died, suggests not only the excruciating pain of cholera but also mirrors popular anxiety about the cadaverization of patient's bodies prior to their death.

Moreover, the coldness of the choleric's body is a corollary of Lélia's refusal of sexual relations that is a common leitmotif throughout the novel. In the first chapter of the second part the narrator observes how the convalescent Lélia is marked by the physical symptoms she previously experienced: 'Tantôt, furtive et discrète, elle passe avec un nerveux frémissement contre des pans de marbre qui la couvrent de leur reflet d'un noir bleuâtre [...] avec une voix qui semble entrecoupée' ['Sometimes, furtively and discreetly, she passes with a nervous shudder against sections of marble which cover her with their bluish-black reflection [...] with a voice which seems broken'].[81] The long shadow of cholera is also felt by the other characters, notably via the motif of Lélia's coldness. Recalling Lélia's 'maladie funeste', Magnus expresses to Sténio a desire to touch her.[82] Later, when again suggesting that he wishes to touch '[les] grands mains effilées, si molles et si belles!' ['her long slender hands, so soft and so beautiful'] of the eponymous heroine, Sténio reinforces the coldness of Lélia's hands, adding 'Et si froides!' ['And so cold!'] to Magnus's description.[83] Here we note the long spectre cast by the

[78] Sand, *Lélia*, p. 60.
[79] Ibid., p. 65.
[80] Ibid., p. 63, 66.
[81] Ibid., p. 74.
[82] Ibid., p. 78.
[83] Ibid., p. 83.

symptomology of cholera: the cold extremities associated with cholera by contemporary medical writers continue to define Lélia after her recovery from the disease. The physical coldness associated with cholera is metaphorized as revealing her sexual frigidity: Lélia's sang froid in the bedside scene is presented as typical of her frosty demeanour and terrifying gaze: 'La figure pâle et le regard méchant et froid de Lélia [...] me pétrifiait' ['The pale face and the evil and cold gaze of Lélia [...] petrified me'].[84] Lélia turns coldness from a symptom of a physical illness into the symptom of a broader social malaise: 'Oh le froid! ce mal pénétrant qui enfonce des aiguilles acérées dans tous les pores! [...] Vous voyez bien que tout se civilise, c'est-à-dire que tout se refroidit. [...] C'est que partout le sang s'appauvrit et se congèle à mesure que l'instinct grandit et se développe'[85] ['Oh the cold! That penetrating pain which digs sharp needles into every pore! [...] You can see that everything is becoming civilized, which is to say that everything is cooling down. [...] Everywhere blood is depleted and frozen as instinct grows and develops'].

In this passage, the novel associates coldness with a resistance to desire and to the constrained gender roles of marriage which is the only socially-sanctioned institution for the fulfilment of female desire. As Waller remarks, Lélia's '*mal du siècle*, far from a crisis in male identity, is largely a symptom of her explicitly feminist discontent'.[86] However, by analysing how Lélia's *mal du siècle* recalls not just generalized malaise or ennui, but also the symptoms of cholera, we can see how, just as cholera renders its victims grotesque and abject, Lélia declares that her refusal of male sexual advances renders her socially and sexually abject: 'La froideur de mes sens me plaçait au-dessous des plus abjectes femmes, l'exaltation de mes pensées m'élevait au-dessus des hommes les plus passionnés' ['The coldness of my senses placed me below the most abject women, the exaltation of my thoughts raised me above the most passionate men'].[87]

Harkness remarks that the motif of Lélia's statuesque coldness is a 'potent symbol not only of the social constraints placed on female subjectivity in the early nineteenth century, but also of the processes of literary signification in which the female character is caught'.[88] Indeed, Lélia's frigidity translates into her transmogrification into a marble statue. The coldness of Lélia's marmoreal body translate into paleness, and she becomes as pallid as a statue. At the opening of the novel, she is described as 'Pâle comme une des statues de marbre blanc qui veillent auprès des

[84] Ibid., p. 86. For frigidity more generally, see Peter Cryle and Alison Moore, *Frigidity: An Intellectual History* (Basingstoke: Palgrave Macmillan, 2011). Duffy explores similar themes of sexual coldness in Zola's *Fécondité*, see Larry Duffy, 'Medical Humanism or *Scientia Sexualis*? Building a Sexological Concept in *Fécondité*', *Nottingham French Studies*, 60 (2021) 317–33.
[85] Sand, *Lélia*, pp. 120–1.
[86] Waller, *The Male Malady*, p. 137.
[87] Sand, *Lélia*, p. 169.
[88] Nigel Harkness, 'Resisting Realist Petrification in George Sand's *Lélia* and Balzac's *Sarrasine*', *French Studies*, 59.2 (2005), 159–72 (p. 68).

tombeaux, vous n'aviez plus rien de terrestre' ['Pale like one of those white marble status that keep watch over tombs, you were no longer of this world'].[89] The whiteness of Lélia herself is extended to include her bedsheets and, via euphemistic metaphor, her status as a virgin. She rests on 'Un lit de satin blanc. Et la vierge de marbre, qui est enchâssée dans la niche de l'est, poussa un profond soupir' ['A bed with white satin. And the marble virgin, enshrined in the eastern niche, let out a deep sigh'].[90] Moreover, it this coldness, or hardness, is responsible for causing physical suffering in those who love her. As Sténio remarks to Lélia: 'Vous êtes froide, Lélia, oh! froide comme le marbre! Moi, je suis mal, je brûle, l'air manque à ma poitrine' ['You are cold, Lélia, oh! Cold like marble! I'm ill, I'm burning, I have no air in my lungs'].[91] The theme of marble also echoes the Pygmalion myth, and Lélia is compared to Galatée in the novel: 'C'est le marbre sans tache de Galatée' ['She is the flawless marble of Galatea'].[92] According to Waller, rewriting the Pygmalion story allows Sand to bring the female statue to life 'not as the perfect object of man's desire, but as a self-contained and troubled subject who rebuffs his self-interested idolization of her'.[93]

However, the marble-esque qualities of Lélia recall not just the Pygmalion myth, but also the corporeal unknowability of cholera. As seen previously, the doctor–patient encounter of *Lélia* specifically draws on the confusion in contemporary medical circles. Although medical writers were generally united on the harrowing symptoms of cholera, marmoreal impenetrability and medical unknowability also characterized contemporary medical discourse about the disease. The *Journal des débats* reflected on the impenetrable mystery of cholera: 'Le monde est bien vieux, dit-on, le monde n'en est pas moins plein de mystères impénétrables. Nos explications ne sont habituellement que l'assimilation d'un phénomène nouveau à un phénomène qui nous est plus familier, mais dont la cause intime nous échappe également' ['The world is very old, they say, yet it is no less full of impenetrable mysteries. Our explanations are usually nothing more than the assimilation of a new addition to a phenomenon which is more familiar to us, but whose root cause escapes us'].[94] For Doctor Tacheron, cholera was unknown and ultimately unknowable in its cause, spread, and treatment: 'Tout ce que nous savons, c'est que la maladie est nouvelle pour nous, redoutable dans ses effets, ignorée dans

89 Sand, *Lélia*, p. 12.
90 Ibid., p. 79.
91 Ibid., p. 216.
92 Ibid., p. 46.
93 Waller, *The Male Malady*, p. 147. For a discussion of Pygmalion and its intersection with the desire of design in Sand, see Harkness, *Men of Their Words*, pp. 136–8. For the Pygmalion myth in nineteenth-century French literature and culture, see Anne Geisler-Szmulewicz, *Le Mythe de Pygmalion au XIXe siècle: pour une approche de la coalescence des mythes* (Paris: Honoré Champion, 1999) and Alexandra Wettlaufer, *Pen vs. Paintbrush: Girodet, Balzac, and the Myth of Pygmalion in Post-Revolutionary France* (New York: Palgrave, 2001).
94 'Rapport sur le choléra-morbus, lu les 26 et 30 juillet, à l'Académie royale de la médecine', *Journal des débats*, 18 February 1832, p. 4.

ses causes et ses modes d'agir' ['All we know is that the disease is new to us, formidable in its effects, yet its causes and modes of action are unknown'].[95] Cholera thus terrorized France in 1832 not just because of its symptomology, but also due to the disease's novelty. Faced with a highly contagious disease that transformed its victims into corpses before doctors' eyes, the medical community found itself perplexed regarding cholera's aetiology and best practices for treatment. It is this medical uncertainty about the choleric body that the novel satirizes during the bedside encounter, again inverting the ordinarily hierarchical doctor–patient relationship.

Sand's *Lélia*, through its references to contemporary medical opinion about cholera's symptoms, pastiches not just the medical tradition but also literary tropes most often identified with Balzac's work. In her ground-breaking analysis of Sand's novels, Schor observes that *La Marquise* is written in response to the *étude de femme* genre as conceived by Balzac. She writes that, in *La Marquise*, 'the cure for women's lack or loss of desire is not, as it is for men who suffer from this syndrome, degrading the object, but in some sense enhancing it through secrecy and illicitness'.[96] The following section expands Schor's brief remark regarding the relationship between Sand's novels and Balzac's *étude de femme* genre in more detail, arguing that *Lélia* responds to the Balzacian *étude de femme* that was a particular literary manifestation of a generalized medical disdain for female bodies. Balzac completed two works whose titles explicitly refer to this genre: the *étude de femme* and the composite novella *Autre étude de femme*.

We have already seen the episodic nature of medicine in *Lélia*, which shows the protagonist's illness in one key scene. In *L'Interdiction*, medicine is equally episodic but even more peripheral to the main plot. *L'Interdiction* revolves around the *juge d'instruction* Jean-Jules Popinot's investigation into the Marquise d'Espard who he suspects is attempting to have her husband declared legally incompetent due to insanity. Rastignac, an urbane dandy rather than the young law student we saw in the Introduction, is in love with the Marquise d'Espard. Having encountered Bianchon in the street when the doctor is on his way to consult with Popinot, Rastignac explains his predicament to him. In *L'Interdiction*, then, we witness an encounter between a doctor and his friend, and it's through his friend's account that Bianchon diagnoses the subject of their conversation, the Marquise. This is an unusual doctor–patient encounter, wherein Rastignac acts as a proxy or stand-in for the Marquise, but one that demonstrates the doctor's authority to construct and master a virtual doctor–patient relationship.

After having listened to Rastignac, Bianchon suspects the Marquise of acting with false intent. To justify his suspicions, Bianchon proclaims that his ability to predict the Marquise's bad intentions comes from the intimate knowledge of the

[95] Tacheron, *Statistique médicale de la mortalité du choléra-morbus*, p. 51.
[96] Schor, *George Sand and Idealism*, p. 48.

human heart that his profession affords him. In a long diatribe against women, Bianchon outlines how medicine allows doctors access to an intimate knowledge of women. Bianchon begins by claiming that he views women only as 'des marionnettes, des poupées et des pantins' ['marionettes, dolls, and puppets'], thus objectifying them and rendering them a sub-human species.[97] The comparison with puppets and dolls also alludes to women's uncanny qualities: although they have superficial human features, they are in fact mechanical duplicates of the human essence. Bianchon evokes the bedside as a locus of secret-sharing: 'Vous passez les nuits à leur chevet [...]; vous avez réussi, vous leur gardez le secret comme si vous étiez mort, elles vous envoient demander votre mémoire et le trouvent horriblement cher' ['You spend nights at their bedside [...]; whenever you succeeded, you keep their secret as if you were dead, they employ you but find your rates frightfully expensive'].[98] Bianchon also compares the role of a doctor to that of a priest, similar to the *médecin-philosophe* analysed in Chapter One, thus transforming the bedside consultation into a confessional scene. Bianchon makes the link between doctor and priest explicit: 'Les médecins sont habitués à juger les hommes et les choses; les plus habiles d'entre nous confessent l'âme en confessant le corps' ['Doctors are used to judging people and things; the most skilful among us confess the soul while confessing the body'].[99] Bianchon claims that, like a priest, the doctor must efface himself to focus solely on the patient. But the doctor's focus is wholly self-serving: by giving the patient the semblance of a beautiful death, and promising to keep their secrets, the doctor can later leverage their influence over the patient in the form of extracting payment.[100]

In response to this tirade, Rastignac remarks that Bianchon must have 'appris bien des choses depuis notre séjour à la Maison Vauquer' ['learnt many things since our stay at the Maison Vauquer'], and indeed Bianchon's callous analysis of the doctor–patient encounter contrasts sharply with a moment in *Le Père Goriot* when, whilst maintaining a vigil at the deathbed of the eponymous character. In that scene, as we saw in the 'Introduction', Bianchon states that that, whilst examining a patient during clinical lessons, unlike his peers at medical school, he always keeps his patients in mind whilst practising medicine. Whereas 'Les médecins qui ont exercé ne voient que la maladie' ['Doctors who have practised see only the

[97] Honoré de Balzac, *Une double famille, suivi du Contrat de mariage et de L'Interdiction*, ed. by Samuel S. de Sacy (Paris: Gallimard, 1973), p. 278.

[98] Ibid., p. 278.

[99] Ibid., p. 277. There is a connection here to Cabanis's model of medicine as discussed in Chapter One.

[100] In *Le Cousin Pons* Bianchon's wealth is a sign of his successful medical practice, as Doctor Poulain remarks: By the time of *Le Cousin Pons*, Bianchon has amassed great wealth to the envy of his less eminent colleagues: 'le docteur Poulain ne pouvait s'empêcher de comparer ses recettes de dix francs dans les jours heureux, à celles de Bianchon, qui vont à cinq ou six cents francs!' ['Doctor Poulain could not help, on good days, comparing his ten-franc receipts to those of Bianchon, which go to five or six hundred francs!']. Honoré de Balzac, *Le Cousin Pons*, ed. by Jacques Thuillier and André Lorant (Paris: Gallimard, 2007), p. 194.

disease'], he claims, but only he continues to see the patient in their entirety, 'moi, je vois encore le malade' ['I still see the patient'].[101] Here Bianchon echoes Foucault's argument that, when an individual patient acquires the status of an object, by being the object rather than the subject of the medical gaze, 'l'application du regard, tour à tour, les éveillera et les fera valoir sur fond d'objectivité' ['the application of the gaze, in turn, will awaken them and make them stand out against a background of objectivity'].[102] Because of this aspect of the medical gaze, Foucault argues, 'Le regard n'est plus réducteur, mais fondateur de l'individu dans sa qualité irréductible' ['The gaze is no longer reductive, but instead creates the individual in his irreducible quality'].[103] In *Le Père Goriot*, then, Bianchon asserts that his medical gaze can affirm and appreciate the patient's singularity. By the time of *L'Interdiction*, however, Bianchon has become much more cynical: although he believes that doctors now perform a similar bedside role to that of priests, he is aware that doctors dissimulate in order to give their patients the impression that their suffering is uniquely beautiful, stating that 'vous exterminez pour leur sauver la plus légère altération de beauté' ['you eclipse yourself to save them the slightest change in their beauty'].[104]

Furthermore, whereas in *Le Père Goriot* Bianchon professes that he can appreciate a patient's individuality, in *L'Interdiction* he becomes more interested in diagnosing and classifying the entire female sex. Bianchon claims that, on account of his medical profession, he can penetrate intimate feminine domestic space. He is thus privy to what he characterizes as the true, monstrous, nature of these women:

> Mon cher, ces femmes de qui vous dites: 'C'est des anges!', moi je les ai vues déshabillées des petites mines sous lesquelles elles couvrent leur âme, aussi bien que des chiffons sous lesquels elles déguisent leurs imperfections: sans manières et sans corset. Elles ne sont pas belles.[105]
> My dear fellow, these women of whom you say: 'They are angels!', I see them stripped of their little façades under which they conceal their souls, as well as the rags under which they disguise their imperfections: without manners and without corsets. They are not beautiful.

It is thus rather surprising, then, Mikhalevitch designates Bianchon as a character who gives to 'la psyché de ses patients (surtout aux femmes) une attention qui le différencie de l'approche purement scientifique et objectiviste de ses plus illustres maîtres et confrères' ['the psyche of his patients (especially to women) an attention which sets him apart from the purely scientific and objective approach

[101] Balzac, *Le Père Goriot*, p. 339.
[102] Foucault, *Naissance de la clinique*, p. 11.
[103] Ibid., pp. 11–12.
[104] Balzac, *L'Interdiction*, p. 278.
[105] Ibid., p. 278.

of his most illustrious masters and colleagues'].[106] Instead, Bianchon characterizes women as monstrous creatures who use the artificial charms of femininity, such as their facial expressions, manners, and corsets to hide what he perceives as their true ugliness. Moreover, rather than making use of his special access to his patients in order to heal them, as we saw for the country doctor in Chapter One, Bianchon uses his intimate knowledge of his female patients to 'diagnose' and identify a *type*, the *femme à la mode* which he considers to be an unnatural specimen since she is ruled by sexual passions rather than by maternal instinct or social conformity: 'La femme à la mode n'est plus une femme: elle est ni mère, ni épouse, ni amante [...] médicalement parlant' ['The *femme à la mode* is no longer a woman: she is neither mother nor wife nor lover [...] medically speaking'].[107] By using his 'qualité de médecin' ['doctor's touch'], Bianchon diagnoses the Marquise as one of these *femmes à la mode*, and warns him of her inevitable temperament: 'Aussi ta marquise a-t-elle tous les symptômes de sa monstruosité, elle a le bec de l'oiseau de proie, l'œil clair et froid, la parole douce; elle est polie comme l'acier d'une mécanique, elle émut tout, moins le cœur' ['Also your Marquise has all the symptoms of her monstrosity, she has the beak of a bird of prey, clear and cold eyes, soft speech; she is polished like the steel of a machine, she touches everything, except the heart'].[108] Later in *L'Interdiction*, Bianchon's suspicions about the Marquise are proved correct as she is revealed to be manipulating her husband in an attempt to steal his fortune. The proxy doctor–patient encounter in this novel, then, points towards the authority of the doctor which is so great that he can correctly diagnose a subject of interest without ever having met them.

The theme of the body, even in a medical context, doubtlessly recalls the question of erotic desire. Desire is intimately tied to narrative and plot, particularly in the nineteenth century: according to Harkness, realist narratives 'function according to a masculine economy of desire, and [...] channels such desire teleologically through a plot which moves inexorably towards climax and resolution'.[109] For Brooks, narratives 'both tell of desire—typically present some story of desire—and arouse and make use of desire as dynamic of signification'.[110] The logic of desire is often channelled through the male gaze: 'Vision is typically a male prerogative, and its object of fascination the woman's body'.[111] Here, plot is produced and driven by heterosexual desire which is sustained through the visual surveillance of the

[106] Mikhalevitch, *Balzac et Bianchon*, p. 299.

[107] Balzac, *L'Interdiction*, p. 279.

[108] Ibid., p. 279. Bianchon's theory espoused in *L'Interdiction* coincides with that of *la femme complète*, described in the following terms in *La Cousine Bette*: '[Ê]tre une honnête et prude femme pour le monde, et se faire courtisane pour son mari' ['[Being] an honest and prudish woman for the world, and becoming a courtesan for her husband']. See Honoré de Balzac, *La Cousine Bette*, ed. by Pierre Barbéris (Paris: Gallimard, 1973), p. 317.

[109] Harkness, *Men of Their Words*, p. 121.

[110] Peter Brooks, *Reading for the Plot: Design and Intention in Narrative* (Cambridge, MA; London: Harvard University Press, 1992), p. 37.

[111] Peter Brooks, *Body Work: Objects of Desire in Modern Narrative* (Cambridge, MA: Harvard University Press, 1993), p. 88.

female body. In this remarkable speech at the beginning of *L'Interdiction*, then, Bianchon creates a paradigm of medicine wherein the doctor's uniquely intimate access to female spaces and bodies a so-called truth about them, thus destroying the myth of their erotic desirability. Bianchon thus weaponizes the medical gaze against women, revealing them as ugly impersonators of femininity and, at the same time, styling the doctor as uniquely positioned to be able to see this supposed truth.

Bianchon's self-proclaimed ability to penetrate women's privacy through intimate knowledge of their bodies recalls Foucault's characterization of the early nineteenth-century scientific turn in medicine and its interest to 'ouvrir quelques cadavres' ['open up some cadavers'].[112] According to Foucault, the increased interest in anatomy was tantamount to the application of the medical gaze onto the interior of the body to reveal its physiological secrets. The anatomical turn meant that medicine began to transcend the previous dichotomy between the external and internal; previously, although doctors would 'read' the body through exterior signs such as taking a patient's pulse and vital signs, the patient's interior body was kept mysterious. Although the popularity of dissection had waxed and waned since the early conception of medicine, Foucault argues that changes in clinical education in the nineteenth century placed a greater emphasis on surgical dissection in the formation of young doctors. Bianchon is a protégé of Desplein, the great surgeon of *La Comédie humaine* modelled on the anatomist and surgeon Guillaume Dupuytren. The medical diatribe of *L'Interdiction* can thus be understood as a similar transcendence of the previous dichotomy between the patient's exterior and interior body, a veritable dissection of the barrier that once separated Bianchon's female patients' external appearance from their internal reality. Paired with Foucault's observation of the erotized vocabulary of the 'couple médecin–malade' mentioned previously, Bianchon's diatribe in *L'Interdiction* can be understood as the sexual-medical penetration of the female patient's body by the male medical gaze (even when that 'gaze' is virtual).

By contrast, in *Lélia*, the medical gaze that appropriates the male gaze and channels its desire into the creation of medical knowledge is rebuffed by the impenetrability of the marmoreal choleric female body. Through its inversion of the Pygmalion myth, Sand's novel questions the male codification of the novel. Although Lélia's marmoreal features no doubt recalls the Pygmalion myth and questions of creative control and freedom, these features' association with the metaphors of cholera symptomology also suggest the intrinsic unknowability of the protagonist. The fragmented opening passages of *Lélia* are instructive in this regard, uniting both Lélia's fundamental unknowability and the pain she provokes, as one of the mysterious opening voices says of her: 'Qui es-tu? et pourquoi ton amour fait-il tant de mal?' ['Who are you? And why does your love hurt me so

[112] The title of chapter seven of Foucault's *Naissance de la clinique*.

much?']. [113] The failure to comprehend Lélia is partly attributed to the failure of external sight—'Plus je vous vois, et moins je vous devine' ['The more I see you, the less I understand you']. [114] In comparison to the penetrating, analytical medical gaze of which Bianchon boasts in *L'Interdiction*, Lélia remains mysteriously enigmatic. Moreover, whereas Bianchon is intent on reducing women to a *type* that represents the entirety of the gender, through her unknowability, Lélia is at once unique and stands as an allegory for the plight of nineteenth-century women. By repelling the knowledge-seeking medical gaze through the frigid metaphors of cholera, Lélia's body becomes both abject and unknowable—a refuge from medical science for a female cholera patient. Instead, Lélia's eyes possess an intense power, which 'brillaient d'un feu sacré' ['shone with a holy fire'] that offers an alternative model of vision and corporeal knowledge and questions the structures of the doctor–patient relationship. [115]

Idealist and Realist Medical Narratives

Balzac's and Sand's differing representations of the doctor–patient relationship and encounter intersect with and shine new light on the literary struggle between realism and idealism in the nineteenth century, thus throwing new light on the relationship between medicine and realism identified by Rothfield and Donaldson-Evans. [116] Schor persuasively argues for the importance of idealism to Sand's œuvre, defining idealism as a form of literary representation that refused to depict the world as it were, and instead depicted a vision of a better world that was morally prescriptive. Schor also highlights that idealism was not rigorously differentiated from realism, and that the two genres can be found in the same piece of work. [117] My analysis of the doctor–patient encounter in *Lélia* contributes to this reading: my comparison of Lélia's condition with contemporary ideas of cholera symptoms demonstrates the extent to which the novel incorporates historical realism. Reboul's characterization of Sand's depiction of cholera as inaccurate and implausible can thus be understood in light of Nancy K. Miller's criticism of Genette:

> The attack on female plots and plausibilities assumes that women cannot or will not obey the rules of fiction. It also assures that the truth devolving from verisimilitude is male. For sensibility, sensitivity, 'extravagance' [...] are taken not merely to be inferior modalities of production but deviation from some obvious truth. [118]

[113] Sand, *Lélia*, p. 7.
[114] Ibid., p. 7.
[115] Ibid., p. 9.
[116] Lawrence Rothfield, *Vital Signs: Medical Realism in Nineteenth-Century Fiction* (Princeton, NJ: Princeton University Press, 1995); Mary Donaldson-Evans, *Medical Examinations: Dissecting the Doctor in French Narrative Prose, 1857–1894* (Lincoln, NE: University of Nebraska Press, 2000).
[117] Schor, *George Sand and Idealism*.
[118] Nancy K. Miller, 'Emphasis Added: Plots and Plausibilities in Women's Fiction', *PMLA*, 96.1 (1981), 36–48 (p. 46).

At the same time, however, *Lélia* engages in idealistic modes insofar as the novel's satire of medicine is a way of imagining a different form of medical encounter and relationship between doctor and patient. More broadly, the 'undecideability or oscillation that violates the laws of generic purity' of Sand's *Lélia* deliberately obscures the linear course of the plot of heterosexual desire most closely associated with the realist novel.[119]

By contrast, when it comes to *L'Interdiction*, a central question is that of narrative 'truth'. The denouement of *L'Interdiction* proves correct Bianchon's initial suspicions about the Marquise d'Espard's bad intentions towards her husband: the Marquise with whom Rastignac tries to start an affair, is in fact a swindler acting under the influence of a malevolent Mesmerist. At stake in predicting the Marquise's true intentions is the nature of truth itself: in response to Bianchon's tirade against women, Rastignac remarks that 'Il y a du vrai dans ce que tu dis' ['There's something true in what you're saying'], to which Bianchon replies 'Du vrai! [...] tout est vrai. Crois-tu donc que je n'aie pas été atteint jusqu'au fond du cœur' ['Some truth! [...] all is true. So do you think that I haven't been struck to the bottom of my heart?'].[120] Bianchon's exclamation in *L'Interdiction* mirrors the famous maxim of the narrator of *Le Père Goriot*: 'ce drame n'est ni une fiction, ni un roman. *All is true*; il est si véritable que chacun peut en reconnaître les éléments chez soi, dans son cœur peut-être' ['This drama is neither a fiction nor a novel. All is true; it is so real that everyone can recognize its elements within themselves, perhaps in their hearts'].[121] As one of the novel's main focalizers, the other being Popinot, with his penetrative medical gaze, Bianchon is thus presented as a guarantor of narrative stability and insight (or even foresight as in Bianchon's case in *L'Interdiction*). Bianchon's narrative reliability is further strengthened by the ways that he is often described in *La Comédie humaine*, possessing an 'air patriarcal, de grands cheveux longs, un front bombé' ['patriarchal air, long hair, a rounded forehead'].[122] Thus, for Félicien Marceau, the doctor is 'le perspicace Bianchon' ['the perceptive Bianchon'] and '[l']un des héros principaux [et] célèbres' ['one of the most important and famous heroes'] of *La Comédie humaine*.[123]

Bianchon also plays an important role as a storyteller in *La Comédie humaine*. In *Autre étude de femme*, Bianchon tells the harrowing tale of 'La Grande Bretèche'. In his story, Madame de Merret's cuckolded husband pressures his wife to swear that their bedroom cupboard is empty, when in fact he knows that her illicit lover is hiding in it. The enraged husband then immediately seals the cupboard by bricking it up, thus dooming the hidden lover to his death. The story ends with the image of Madame de Merret remaining in her room for days whilst listening to

119 Schor, *George Sand and Idealism*, p. 59.
120 Balzac, *L'Interdiction*, p. 279.
121 Balzac, *Le Père Goriot*, p. 22.
122 Honoré de Balzac, *La Muse du département; Un prince de la bohème*, ed. by Patrick Berthier (Paris: Gallimard, 2007), p. 76.
123 See Félicien Marceau, *Balzac et son monde* (Paris: Gallimard, 1986), p. 122.

the pained groans of her lover who slowly starves to death from behind the wall. The doctor details how the mysterious house and its accompanying ghoulish tale which

> me laissa en proie à des pensées vagues et ténébreuses, à une curiosité romanesque, à une terreur religieuse assez semblable au sentiment profond qui nous saisit quand nous entrons à la nuit dans une église sombre où nous apercevons une faible lumière lointaine sous les arceaux élevés; une figure indécise glisse, un frottement de robe ou de soutane se fait entendre... nous avons frissonné.[124]

> leaves me prey to vague and dark thoughts, to a romantic curiosity, to a religious terror similar to the deep feeling that seizes us when, at night, we enter a dark church in which we perceive a distant, weak light under the high arches; an indistinct face half appears, we hear the friction of a dress or a cassock... we shivered.

The tale, by relying on the narrative techniques of the *roman policier*, establishes Bianchon as a mystery-solver in addition to a master storyteller with strong links to the narration of *La Comédie humaine* itself. Indeed, as D. A. Miller observes regarding *Une ténébreuse affaire*, 'Like Balzac's doctors and lawyers, [the police spies Peyrade and Corentine are] privy to what goes on behind the "scènes de la vie privée", and they thus resemble the novelist whose activity is also conceived as a penetration of social surfaces.'[125]

Furthermore, 'La Grande Bretèche' establishes Bianchon as an intradiegetic storyteller, within the world of *La Comédie humaine* itself. As the Duc de Rhétoré says in *Autre étude de femme*, 'Les histoires que conte le docteur [...] font des impressions profondes [...] mais douces' ['The stories that the doctor recounts [...] create deep but pleasant impressions'].[126] Bianchon's investigations of the abandoned house, leading him to uncover the wife's infidelity and her lover's murder, are thus transformed by the *mise en abyme* into the doctor's opportunity to prove his talents as a storyteller elsewhere in *La Comédie humaine*. The power of Bianchon's story allows him to influence the physical movements of his female interlocuters, again displaying the doctor's power over women: 'toutes les femmes se levèrent de table, et le charme sous lequel Bianchon les avait tenus fut dissipé par ce mouvement' ['All the women rose from the table, and the charm under which Bianchon had held them was dissipated by this movement'].[127] The fact that Bianchon narrates

[124] Honoré de Balzac, *Les Secrets de la princesse de Cadignan et autres études de femme*, ed. by Samuel S. de Sacy and Jean Roudaut (Paris: Gallimard, 1980), p. 105.

[125] D. A. Miller, *The Novel and the Police* (Berkeley, CA; London: University of California Press, 1988), p. 23.

[126] Balzac, *Autres étude de femme*, p. 89.

[127] Ibid., p. 114.

both of Balzac's works which bear the name of the genre, the *Étude de femme* and *Autre étude de femme*, thus suggests the medical profession's unique intimacy with, and insight into, the sordid lives of women. *L'Interdiction* and the accompanying *études de femme* narrated by Bianchon paint a picture of the commanding male medical gaze that penetrates and understands women's bodies, facilitating his powers as a narrator. At the apogee of his career then, Bianchon becomes a self-confessed researcher and narrator of the (female) body.

At least part of Bianchon's narratorial authority is therefore derived from the relationship that he has with his patients, affording him intimate access into the most private and secret areas of his patient's lives. Although this access and authority grants Bianchon a degree of power over his patients, the bilateral nature of the doctor–patient relationship means that Bianchon is profoundly shaped by his medical interactions. We see such an effect most clearly in *La Muse du département*, which features a Bianchon at the apogee of his medical career. At the moment of his arrival in Sancerre, Bianchon is repeatedly declared a man of superior moral, social, and professional standing, particularly in comparison to Dinah de La Baudraye: he is a 'savant interprète de la nature humaine' ['a wise interpreter of human nature'] and a 'lion' ['king'] of Parisian society.[128] Dinah, despite her local popularity is a poor rival to the real George Sand, as the narrator sardonically quips: 'On se passionna, dans l'arrondissement de Sancerre, pour Madame de La Baudraye, en qui l'on voulut voir la future rivale de George Sand' ['In the arrondissement of Sancerre, people were enthralled by Madame de La Baudraye, in whom they wanted to see a future rival of George Sand'].[129] Harbouring a secret love for Dinah, which goes unsaid in the novel yet is nonetheless detected by Dinah, his medical vocation prevents her from imagining a relationship between them. For Dinah, all encounters with Bianchon recall the clinical doctor–patient encounter and thus preclude romantic feeling: 'elle pensait aux devoirs de la profession et se demandait si une femme pouvait jamais être autre chose qu'un *sujet* aux yeux d'un médecin qui voit tant de *sujets* dans sa journée!' ['she thought of his profession's duties and asked herself if a woman could ever be anything other than a *subject* in the eyes of a doctor who saw many *subjects* over the course of his day'].[130] This foreclosure of romantic feeling for the doctor extends to the failure of Bianchon's erotic desirability: later in the novel, Bianchon's scientific coolness means that the touch of his hand awakens nothing in her.[131] For Dinah,

[128] Balzac, *La Muse du département*, p. 87. Andrew Counter observes that similar phrases for Juge Popinot are undermined by their hyperbole: indeed, it is Bianchon who remarks that Popinot 'est juge comme la mort est la mort' ['is a judge like death is death']. I would venture that critics who take this portrayal of Popinot seriously are doing so due to their implicit faith in Bianchon as a morally upstanding character. See Andrew Counter, '*L'Interdiction*, or, Balzac on the Margins of Law and Realism', *Law and Humanities*, 11.1 (2017), 24–43 (p. 39).

[129] Balzac, *La Muse du département*, pp. 87, 70.

[130] Ibid., p. 139; original emphasis.

[131] Ibid., p. 146.

the cold professional nature with which the doctor conducts an otherwise intimate encounter with women's bodies forecloses any erotic interest between them. Bianchon's encounters with his patients forestall the development of his romantic relationships.

If Sand's *Lélia* obscures male heterosexual desire and thus the motors of realist plot, the failure of Bianchon's desire in *La Muse du département* also raises questions about the supposed narrative power of Balzac's favoured medical character. Brooks argues that the hero of the nineteenth-century French novel should be understood as a 'desiring machine' whose presence in the novel 'creates and sustains a narrative of movement through the forward march of desire, projecting the self onto the world through scenarios of desire imagined and then acted upon.'[132] The failure of Bianchon's desire for Dinah is thus tantamount to the threatened failure of plot itself. The reason for this forestalling is, paradoxically, Bianchon's medical profession. On the one hand, as seen in *L'Interdiction*, Bianchon's medical profession gains him access to his patient's most intimate secrets and, in the case of the Marquise d'Espard, knowledge of these secrets allows Bianchon to trigger the main plot by planting seeds of doubt in Rastignac's mind. On the other hand, in *La Muse du département*, it is Bianchon's profession that proves a turn-off for Dinah. Although his role as a doctor gains him access to plot and the desires of others, it forestalls his own. The foreclosure of Bianchon's desires due to his chosen profession perhaps explains the character's psychological blankness that scholars observe.[133] I would add to this remark that this nexus of failed desire and plot explains Bianchon's peripherality in *La Comédie humaine*: as a doctor his presence is largely required only when characters fall sick. Although his medical knowledge renders Bianchon an essential attendee at pivotal sickbed and deathbed scenes, affording him glimpses into the reality of nineteenth-century life as he boasts in *L'Interdiction*, ultimately *La Comédie humaine* finds this to be an impoverished narratorial perspective that sees the doctor embroiled in ethical questions that tarnish the extent to which he can be considered a moral anchor of the novelistic cycle.[134]

Finally, the failure of Bianchon's desire and his own romantic plotline allows us to re-read his telling of 'La Grande Bretèche'. The story reappears in *La Muse du département* when guests take turns recounting stories following a dinner. Bianchon repeats the story of 'La Grande Bretèche' again, to supposedly great acclaim: 'Ce fut d'ailleurs la même perfection dans les gestes, dans les intonations qui valut tant d'éloges au docteur chez mademoiselle des Touches quand il la raconta pour

[132] Brooks, *Reading for the Plot*, pp. 39–40.

[133] See Marceau, *Balzac et son monde*, p. 259.

[134] Although the narrator insists on Bianchon's 'franchise, [...] la bonhomie' and 'sa profession', Diana Knight comments on the doctor's entanglement in less than professionally ethical practices in *La Muse du département*. See Diana Knight, 'Conjugal Secrets in Balzac's *La Muse du département*', *Nineteenth-Century French Studies*, 40.3–4 (2012), 273–86.

la première fois' ['Moreover, it was the same perfection of gestures and intonation that earned the doctor so much praise at Mademoiselle des Touches's house when he told it for the first time'], producing the same effect on his interlocuters. Thus 'Le dernier tableau du Grand d'Espagne mourant de faim et debout dans l'armoire où l'a muré le mari de Madame de Merret [...] produisit tout son effet' ['The last image of the Spanish grandee, dying of hunger and standing in the cupboard walled up by the husband of Madame de Merret [...] had all the desired effect'] since there was 'un moment de silence assez flatteur pour Bianchon' ['a moment of silence for Bianchon that was fairly flattering'].[135] Whereas Bianchon's earlier recountings of 'La Grande Bretèche' testified to his success as a narrator, in this instance the narrator's sardonic comment that the anecdote allowed Bianchon a moment of appreciation that was merely 'assez flatteur' ['fairly flattering']. The ambivalence of the 'moment de silence' could perhaps be understood as hinting at a second meaning. Bianchon's interlocutors could be stunned into silence, but the silence could equally be seen as a knowing, awkward one that mutely acknowledges Bianchon's narrative failure, on which even the narrator themselves dare not comment.[136]

Conclusion

Sand's *Lélia* overturns the hierarchical nature of the doctor–patient relationship by critiquing medicine's claim to control over the illness narrative through positivistic science and rejecting the doctor's attempts to understand the patient's body. The novel achieves this via a doctor–patient encounter in which the patient criticizes the ideal of a good doctor–patient relationship itself. Sand uses the medical vocabulary of the 1832 cholera epidemic to express these themes in *Lélia*'s bedside scene. Cholera, as a potent generator of myth, is used by Sand to articulate scepticism about the medical profession as well as the abject status of the female body. Furthermore, we have seen that Sand's novel is influenced by, and criticizes, ideas found within Balzac's *La Peau de chagrin* and the *étude de femme* genre. Sand borrows the polyphony of the earlier novel's bedside scene but criticizes Balzac's redemptive 'good' doctor. Cholera is essential to Sand's project here: the 1832 epidemic provides the medical and physical vocabulary through which Sand builds on and parodies Balzac's novel. Looking more broadly at *La Comédie humaine*, Bianchon's position in the Balzacian *étude de femme*, as a

135 Balzac, *La Muse du département*, p. 100.

136 Bianchon's companion in Sancerre, Étienne Lousteau, as a journalist, also shares a connection with Balzac *qua* author, and Bianchon and Lousteau jostle for both narrative power and sexual power over Dinah throughout the novel suggesting a struggle between medico-realist narrative strategies and Romantic-idealist strategies. For a similar reading of *L'Interdiction*, see Counter, '*L'Interdiction*, or, Balzac on the Margins of Law and Realism'.

knower of women and a narrator of tales about them, is also resisted in *Lélia* through the eponymous heroine's unknowability and physical impenetrability. These themes are well established in scholarship about Sand, but this chapter has established the extent to which Sand relies on the medical discourse of cholera to articulate the extent to which Lélia cannot be known by her male admirers. Overall, *Lélia* claims the bedside scene and the patient's body as belonging to Lélia alone, rather than to her doctor or penetrating *regard médical*. Furthermore, the doctor–patient encounter is at the heart of Sand's criticism of Balzac's idealized medical man since the Balzacian medical encounter presumes an all-powerful doctor and a submissive patient on which realism, as well as its discontents, was founded.

In *La Peau de chagrin*, the conventional binary between doctor and patient during the bedside encounter is replaced with a polyphony of doctors' voices. Medicine is satirized but ultimately redeemed through Bianchon's humanism. In *L'Interdiction*, we see a virtual doctor–patient encounter, wherein Bianchon encounters the patient only through his chance (and narratively peripheral) meeting with Rastignac. Despite Bianchon's interest in what is termed as truth, the doctor has an ambiguous relationship with realist narration in *La Comédie humaine*, perhaps suggesting a less that straightforward analogy between medicine and realism in the nineteenth-century novel. Sand's *Lélia* subverts the hierarchal relationship between doctor and patient in the novel's dramatic encounter, questioning the foundation of the Balzacian doctor's authority.

Finally, reading Sand's *Lélia* as a pastiche of *La Peau de chagrin* and the Balzacian *étude de femme* throws new light on the literary relationship between the two authors. Balzac's parodies of Sand are well known: Félicité des Touches is a thinly veiled portrait of her, and Dinah de La Baudraye is a more exaggerated parody of the *type* of the female writer. Yet Sand rewrites the character that will become known as the 'astre' of *La Comédie humaine* by parodying Bianchon in *Lélia*. Indeed, in the preface to the 1841 novel *Horace*, in which the eponymous character is a law student in Paris, the occupation of Bianchon's double, Rastignac, Sand appropriates Balzac's discourse of *type* and truth: 'Horace représente un type moderne très-fidèle et très-répandu' ['Horace represents a very faithful and widespread modern stock character'].[137]

[137] George Sand, *Horace* (Paris: Hetzel et Cie; Victor Lecou, 1854), p. 1.

Chapter Four
Zola's *Lourdes* and the Mysteriousness of the Doctor–Patient Relationship

Introduction

Throughout this study, we have seen how the doctor–patient relationship in the nineteenth-century French novel broadens conventional definitions of illness. In these texts, illness and healing can include the local vicinity (Chapter One); can be imitated and performed disease (Chapter Two); and can generate new forms of metaphor and narrative (Chapter Three). In this chapter we turn our attention to how this enlarged understanding of illness puts the doctor–patient relationship under further pressure in the late nineteenth century, particularly in response to advances in microbiology. I demonstrate how Zola's *Lourdes* illustrates that the doctor–patient relationship should preserve its centrality to the modern medical experience by embracing what is unknown and the unknowable about illness. The central theme of the novel is the enigmatic nature of the ill body and the novel circles around how best to approach, understand, and heal this condition. To a certain extent, this healing is framed as occurring through a conventionally hierarchical doctor–patient relationship wherein the doctor embodies the penetrating medical gaze. Rothfield observes that medical discourse of observation and penetration was inserted into the nineteenth-century novel as literary and narratological paradigms, with the result that the relationship between author and text is modelled on that between doctors and patients.[1] But in this chapter I want to go beyond this analogous relationship between medicine and literature by suggesting that, in Zola's novel *Lourdes*, the doctor–patient relationship is presented as a central component in the re-imagining of medical science in the late nineteenth century. Although the reader may expect that medicine came closer towards our twenty-first-century understanding of a 'scientific' field following the revolution in microbiology during the 1850s, in this chapter I illustrate how *Lourdes* depicts a form of medicine that in fact embraces the mysteriousness of scientific medicine. Zola's novel proposes an alternative approach to medicine by proposing a new form of healing relationship that goes beyond the confines and limitations of what we have so far seen within the doctor–patient relationship.

[1] Lawrence Rothfield, *Vital Signs: Medical Realism in Nineteenth-Century Fiction* (Princeton: Princeton University Press, 1995), p. 37.

The Doctor–Patient Relationship and the Nineteenth-Century French Novel. Sarah Jones, Oxford University Press.
 DOI: 10.1093/oso/9780198893790.003.0005

Zola's *Lourdes* is the first novel of the triptych *Les Trois Villes*, composed at a similar time to *Le Docteur Pascal* and published in the year following the conclusion of the *Rougon-Macquart* cycle. The novel follows Pierre Froment, a priest who has lost his faith in religion, and Marie de Guersaint, a paralysed young woman who (the novel suggests) is suffering from hysteria, on a pilgrimage to Lourdes. The novel is divided into five sections corresponding to a different day that Marie and Pierre spend at Lourdes. Each section is divided into five chapters, and the final chapter is organized around a character relating the story of Bernadette Soubirous, the shepherdess whose visions of the Virgin Mary between February and July 1858 led to the foundation of the Grotto and the establishment of Lourdes as a pilgrimage destination for the sick. The novel returns tirelessly to the enigmatic aspects of health, medicine, and belief, asking how the patient can be healed through trust and feeling. The mysterious nature of healing is central to how *Lourdes* associates the seemingly disparate phenomena of hysteria and microbiological science. Zola's novel demonstrates the idea that medicine must use the ambiguities of the doctor–patient relationship to encompass these invisible, apparently inexplicable phenomena. The risk would be, according to *Lourdes*, that these phenomena continue to be claimed by organized religion, characterized as threatening procreation with its cult of virginal sterility. The novel thus suggests the extent to which the doctor–patient relationship should prioritize compassion above all else. Like *Le Docteur Pascal*, *Lourdes* grapples with questions at the intersection between faith and medicine.[2] Rather than advocating a scientific conception of experimental medicine, as may be anticipated given the ideas Zola expressed in 'Le Roman expérimental', *Lourdes* focuses on, and valorizes, doctor–patient relationships in which the doctor embraces the mysterious forces that act on the body in the forms of hysterical paralysis and microbes. Further, the novel moves beyond the hierarchical and role-defined nature of the doctor–patient relationship in order to consider a broader form of healing relationship that is better placed to respond to the myriad ways that illness can develop and effect those it afflicts.

There are a number of ethical considerations that arise when discussing *Lourdes* from the perspective of medicine and illness. Like the novels analysed in Chapter One, *Lourdes* idealizes medicine as a force that can right some of the perceived wrongs of the modern world, namely what Zola saw as the undue influence of the Catholic Church on France's moral and sexual life. *Lourdes* thus has a clearly defined agenda: as a *roman à these* it attempts to explore the psychosomatic and socio-cultural origin of miracles. The novel's overall conclusion is that Catholicism's interest in miracles emanates from its veneration of human suffering, and it presents medicine as an antidote to this nefarious influence. But whilst it styles medical science as a paternal, benevolent attempt to

[2] Jacques Noiray, 'Préface' in Émile Zola, *Lourdes*, ed. by Jacques Noiray (Paris: Gallimard, 1995), pp. 7–27 (p. 7).

rescue young women from the Church, the novel's focalization through the religious sceptic Pierre silences female characters' voices and experiences. In this way, the novel replicates the hierarchical and asymmetric power dynamic integral to the conventional doctor–patient relationship trope. In this chapter, I take these features into account whilst also exploring the centrality that *Lourdes* gives to the doctor–patient relationship in the context of fin-de-siècle France. However, I demonstrate that *Lourdes* is not just a *roman à these*,[3] but, like *Le Médecin de campagne*, it contains elements that dissent from the novel's overall stance, such as criticism of the portrayal of the female body, gender roles, and disability.

Medical Encounters and Hysteria

The group portrait 'Une leçon clinique à la Salpêtrière' ['A Clinical Lesson at the Salpêtrière'] by Pierre Aristide André Brouillet depicts Jean-Martin Charcot demonstrating hypnosis on a hysterical patient who lies helpless in the arms of Doctor Joseph Babinski. At the same time, Charcot lectures to a group of male physicians. In this image, the female patient is an object of scientific study in addition to a site of medical domination. Now hypnotized, her limp body is decentred from the image which instead focuses on Charcot, who asserts his absolute command over both the patient and his eager interlocuters. Analysing Charcot's photographs of hysterical patients, Didi-Huberman similarly argues that the doctor's control of both the patient's body and the production of their image assured his own authority over his subjects of study.[4] *Lourdes* depicts two seemingly comparable encounters between Marie and her doctors. The first is narrated through Pierre, and recounts Marie's various encounters with medical professionals that have led her to travel to the healing waters at Lourdes. The second occurs when she enters the *bureau des constatations médicales* ['medical office'], whose doctors will decide whether or not her cure should be declared as miraculous.

Marie's first doctor–patient encounters are recounted through the narrative frame of Pierre's own memories of the consultations, accessed through Zola's quintessential use of free indirect discourse. On the long train journey from Paris to Lourdes, Pierre reflects on the doctor–patient encounters which led him and

[3] See, for example, René Ternois, *Zola et son temps: Lourdes, Rome, Paris*, (Paris: Belles lettres, 1961), pp. 213–49.

[4] Georges Didi-Huberman, *Invention de l'hystérie: Charcot et l'iconographie photographique de la Salpêtrière* (Paris: Macula, 1982), pp. 17–31. As Elaine Showalter observes, Charcot was known for 'his probing gaze that seemed to penetrate [...] to the heart of the patient'. See Elaine Showalter, 'Hysteria, Feminism, and Gender', in Sander L. Gilman, Helen King, Roy Porter, G. S. Rousseau, and Elaine Showalter, *Hysteria Beyond Freud* (Berkeley, CA: University of California Press, 1993), p. 309.

Marie to embark on the pilgrimage. His memories serve as the basis of the main narrative of the chapter of the novel's first section. Confined to a wheelchair for a decade, Marie and her family desperately sought medical advice as to the nature of, and potential cure for, her otherwise inexplicable paralysis. Although the journey to Lourdes had already been decided upon, Pierre hurriedly arranges for a final medical examination for her: 'Pierre avait exigé une dernière consultation de Médecins, pour savoir si Marie était réellement transportable' ['Pierre had asked for a final medical consultation to know if Marie was really able to travel'].[5] The narrator remarks that, during these consultations, 'c'était là encore une scène qui s'évoquait, dont il revoyait certains détails avec persistance, tandis que d'autres s'effaçaient déjà' ['it was then that another scene was conjured up, some of the details of which he was seeing again and again, whilst other details were already fading'], positioning Pierre's memories as the central narrative frame for this episode. Pierre remembers two doctors who had treated Marie in the past, 'l'un croyant à une rupture des ligaments larges, l'autre diagnostiquant une paralysie due à une lésion de la moelle' ['one believing in a rupture of the broad ligament, the other diagnosing paralysis caused by a lesion of the spinal cord'], but that they nevertheless decide on a vague diagnosis, 'cette paralysie, avec des accidents, peut-être, du côté des ligaments' ['this paralysis, with perhaps some accident having occurred to her ligaments'].[6] This diagnosis is enough for them to approve Marie's trip to Lourdes, as well as to reassure Pierre, 'Cela devait déterminer Pierre, car il trouvait ces messieurs très prudents, très soucieux de la vérité' ['This helped Pierre make up his mind, since he found these men very cautious and very concerned with the truth'].[7]

After reflecting on Marie's encounter with the Parisian doctors, Pierre recounts the final doctor–patient encounter before the group's departure for Lourdes. The consultation is with a doctor named Beauclair, a distant cousin of Pierre. He asks about Marie's father, 'cet architecte [...] à l'esprit faible' ['this architect [...] with a weak mind'] in line with Zola's interest in *Les Rougon-Marquart* on the effects of familial hereditary.[8] Beauclair delicately examines his patient, after which he reaches a diagnosis of ovarian dysfunction: 'il s'était assuré, en la palpant, discrètement, que la douleur avait fini par se localiser à l'ovaire gauche' ['he made sure, by palpating discreetly, that the pain had eventually settled on the left ovary'].[9] Marie's pain moves around her body when the doctor applies pressure to the ovaries: 'lorsqu'on appuyait là, cette douleur semblait remonter vers la gorge, en une masse lourde qui l'étouffait' ['when that area was pressed, the pain

[5] Zola, *Lourdes*, p. 67.
[6] Ibid., p. 67.
[7] Ibid., p. 67.
[8] Ibid., p. 67.
[9] Ibid., p. 67.

seemed to go up towards the throat, in a heavy mass that choked her']. [10] In this medical encounter, Beauclair has a physical connection with his patient's body that leads to the ability to provoke symptoms through his touch.

The doctor–patient relationship depicted in this scene, particularly the attention placed on Marie's ovaries, is reminiscent of that between hysteria patients and their doctors during the nineteenth century. Charcot coined the term *zones hystérogènes* to suggest how areas of the body, particularly the female reproductive organs, were focal points for the symptoms of hysteria, described as 'des régions du corps plus ou moins circonscrites, au niveau desquelles la pression où le simple frottement détermine, plus ou moins rapidement, le phénomène de l'aura, auquel succède quelquefois, si l'on insiste, l'attaque hystérique' ['regions of the body more or less circumscribed, where pressure or simple friction causes, more or less rapidly, the aura phenomenon, which is sometimes followed by a hysterical attack']. [11] Charcot goes on to explain how applying and relieving pressure to the *zones hystérogènes* can control the patient's symptoms, effectively allowing the doctor to control his patient's body: 'Ces points, ou mieux ces plaques, ont encore la propriété d'être le siège d'une sensibilité permanente [...]. L'attaque, une fois développée, peut être souvent arrêtée au moyen d'une pression énergique exercée sur ces mêmes points' ['These points, or rather these plates, still have the property of being the seat of a permanent sensitivity [...]. The attack, once developed, can often be stopped by means of energetic pressure exerted on these same points']. [12] Charcot links the physical position and biological role of a woman's reproductive organs to an ongoing illness and casts himself as able to cure such disturbances through touch alone.

Although Beauclair is not explicitly characterized as a proponent of Charcot's theories, the parallels with the new science of hysteria are self-evident. Furthermore, given Zola's meticulous research for *Les Rougon-Macquart*, Thompson maintains that Zola would have conducted thorough medical reading for *Lourdes*. [13] *Lourdes* also reconstructs the asymmetric doctor–patient relationship imagined by Charcot: Beizer points out that Charcot's emphasis on the hysterogenic zones maintains the theme of the biologically predetermined notion of feminine character and role, and thus were tantamount to a medical disciplining of the hysteric's body through the doctor–patient relationship. [14] Of course, as we saw in the

[10] Ibid., p. 67.
[11] Jean-Martin Charcot, *Leçons sur les maladies du système nerveux*, 3 vols (Paris: Lecrosnieret Babé, 1890), III, p. 88.
[12] Ibid., p. 88.
[13] Hannah Thompson, *Taboo: Corporeal Secrets in Nineteenth-Century France* (Oxford: Legenda, 2013), p. 51. For Zola's research for *Les Rougon-Macquart*, see Cabanès, *Le Corps et la maladie dans les récits réalistes*, pp. 241–3. For Zola's research on the history of Lourdes and the biography of Bernadette, see Ternois, *Zola et son temps*, pp. 320–1.
[14] Janet L. Beizer, *Ventriloquized Bodies: Narratives of Hysteria in Nineteenth-Century France* (Ithaca, NY: Cornell University Press, 1994), p. 7.

'Introduction', hysteria is a key avenue of inquiry in nineteenth-century French studies' interest in representations of medicine. These analyses are often productively linked to questions of power and gender: Matlock, for example, highlights how transgressions of the social and sexual order demonstrate that sexual deviants, such as the prostitute and the hysteric, become 'privileged objects of knowledge in [their] own right' and are attacked by those who cast them as deviants.[15] However, this power dynamic is not dominated by the doctor alone, as my analysis of *Lamiel* and *Lélia* demonstrated in Chapters Two and Three. Didi-Huberman thus asserts the hysterical patient's ability to manipulate her doctor, regardless of the latter's scientific and professional authority: 'À la Salpêtrière [...] les hystériques n'ont pas cessé de faire de l'œil à leurs médecins. Ce fut une espèce de loi du genre, non seulement la loi du fantasme hystérique (désir de captiver), mais encore la loi de toute l'institution asilaire elle-même' ['At the Salpêtrière [...] the hysterics did not stop making eyes at their doctors. It was a kind of law of its kind, not only the law of the hysterical fantasy (the desire to captivate) but also the law of the entire asylum itself'].[16] The new science of hysteria, its medical practitioners, and its institutions, worked to control and correct the bodies of the women diagnosed as hysterical. The attention paid by Beauclair to Marie's ovaries through his emphasis on physical examination suggests that Beauclair can be understood from the perspective of the new medicine of hysteria and the hierarchical doctor–patient relationship that it depended on and perpetuated.

Lourdes also draws on an idealized conception of Mesmerism, a predecessor of Charcot's concept of hysteria. Tracing the history of medicine's attempt to solve the enigma of the link between body and mind, the medical historian Henri Ellenberger states that 'the development of modern dynamic psychiatry can be traced to Mesmer's animal magnetism'.[17] Like Mesmer, and unlike Charcot whose *leçons du mardi* were well known and well attended by both physicians and the general public, Beauclair, despite his 'vive intelligence' ['lively intelligence'], is 'encore peu connu et [...] bizarre' ['still little known and [...] strange'].[18] Animal magnetism referred to an invisible natural force possessed by all living beings and which was responsible for their health and well-being: Mesmer stated that 'Un fluide universellement répandu [...] et qui, de sa nature, est susceptible de recevoir, propager et communiquer toutes les impressions du movement, est le moyen de

[15] Jann Matlock, *Scenes of Seduction: Prostitution, Hysteria, and Reading Difference in Nineteenth-Century France* (New York: Columbia University Press, 1994), p. 3.

[16] Didi-Huberman, *Invention de l'hystérie*, p. 168.

[17] Henri F. Ellenberger, *The Discovery of the Unconscious: The History and Evolution of Dynamic Psychiatry* (London: Fontana, 1994), p. 69. Adam Crabtree similarly contends that eighteenth- and nineteenth-century research into animal magnetism 'led directly to the evolution of a new paradigm for understanding the nature of the human psyche and mental disturbance: the alternate-consciousness paradigm [which] opened up the possibility of an intrapsychic cause of mental disturbance, pointing to the influence of unconscious mental activity as the source of unaccountable thoughts or impulses'. See Adam Crabtree, *From Mesmer to Freud: Magnetic Sleep and the Roots of Psychological Healing* (New Haven, CT; London: Yale University Press, 1993), p. vii.

[18] Zola, *Lourdes*, p. 67. Laurence Brockliss and Colin Jones, *The Medical World of Early Modern France* (Oxford: Clarendon Press, 1997), pp. 783–801.

cette influence' ['A fluid that is universally present [...] and that, because of its nature, can receive, propagate, and communicate all the impressions of movement and the means of this influence'].[19] This fluid is so critical to life, he argues, that all illnesses are caused by interruptions in its flow around the body. Understanding how the universal fluid functions thus allows the doctor to heal any patient: 'le médecin jugera sûrement l'origine, la nature, et les progrès des maladies, même des plus compliquées; il en empêchera l'accroissement, et parviendra à leur guérison, sans jamais exposer le malade à des effets dangereux ou des suites fâcheuses, quel que soient l'âge, le tempérament et le sexe' ['the doctor will judge with certainty the origin, nature, and progress of illnesses, even the most complicated ones; he will prevent their worsening and bring about their cure, without ever exposing the patient to dangerous effects or unfortunate consequences, whatever their age, temperament, or sex'].[20] By understanding animal magnetism, the doctor thus masters the domaine of medicine and is able to control both the effect of medication and even the nature of illness itself: 'Qu'avec son secours, le médecin est éclairé sur l'usage des médicamens; qu'il perfectionne leur action, et qu'il provoque et dirige les crises salutaires, de manière à s'en rendre le maître' ['With his help, the doctor is enlightened on the use of medication; he perfects its action, and he provokes and directs beneficial outbreaks in such a way as to make himself master of them'].[21] It is telling that, in Mesmer's description of healing, or the 'dernière perfection' ['final perfection'] of medicine, the patient is reduced to a vessel of disease or medication that the doctor can control at whim.[22] The *rapport* between Mesmerist and patient is thus one of domination and submission, but also of co-presence, perception, and painless intervention: the Mesmerist heals his patient thanks to his physical presence near their body, allowing him to perceive the blockages of universal fluid, and subsequently work to remove them without causing further harm. I will discuss the erotic dimension of these encounters later, but my point here is to foreground the extent to which Mesmer uses the language of the *rapport* to suggest a non-invasive path to the end of physical and mental pain, thus placing the doctor–patient encounter squarely in the centre of a patient's healing process. Building on contemporary medical discourse surrounding hysteria, itself rooted in eighteenth-century Mesmerism, the doctor–patient encounters recounted at the beginning of *Lourdes* foreground similar elements to that in Charcot's and Mesmer's approach to medicine: namely, that physical proximity between doctor and patient, and the unique relationship that they develop between themselves due to this, helps facilitate an understanding of a patient's illness as well as potential cures.

Mesmer, Charcot, and Zola's Beauclair are united by a belief that medicine should embrace the mysterious aspects of illness to alleviate patients' symptoms. Despite the physical manifestation of Marie's paralysis, Beauclair maintains that

[19] Franz Anton Mesmer, *Mémoire sur la découverte du magnétisme animal* (Genève: Didot, 1779), p. 74.
[20] Ibid., p. 81
[21] Ibid., p. 81
[22] Ibid., p. 83.

the non-physical cause of her condition means that she can be cured by her own will: 'il s'était écrié qu'il fallait la mener à Lourdes, qu'elle y serait sûrement guérie, si elle était certaine de l'être' ['he declared that she should be brought to Lourdes, that she would surely be cured there if she was certain it would happen'] since 'la foi suffisait' ['faith was enough'].[23] Here Beauclair suggests that, if Marie believes in miracles, then she will be cured by one. Beauclair gestures towards two historical cases of his: 'deux de ses clients, très pieuses, envoyées par lui l'année auparavant, étaient revenues éclatantes de santé' ['two of his very pious clients, sent by him the year before, had returned radiantly healthy'].[24] Beauclair's statement resonates with work that Charcot first begun in 1892, two years before *Lourdes* was published. Charcot claimed that, due to the mysterious intermingling of body and mind, the belief in miraculous healing could precipitate its occurrence in the most devout hysterical patients: 'La guérison, [...] produit direct de la *faith-healing*, que l'on appelle communément en thérapeutique du nom de miracle est, on peut le démontrer dans la majorité des cas, un phénomène naturel' ['The healing, the direct product of faith-healing, which is commonly called a miracle by therapy, can be demonstrated in the majority of cases to be a natural phenomenon'][25] The two main requirements for such a miracle are a particular patient disposition and a particular relationship with the body: 'le domaine de la *faith-healing* est limité; pour produire ses effets, elle doit s'adresser à des cas dont la guérison n'exige aucune autre intervention que cette puissance que possède l'esprit sur le corps' ['the realm of faith-healing is limited; to be effective, it must address cases where healing requires no intervention other than this power of the mind over the body'].[26] In short, Charcot claimed that miracles can heal physical symptoms because of the extent to which the underlying illness may have an emotional or mental cause. For these reasons, Beauclair 'refusa absolument de signer un certificat' ['outright refused to sign a medical certificate'] since the doctor rebuffs the suggestion that Marie's paralysis has a wholly physical cause.[27] As we will see, this first medical encounter profoundly shapes the scene in the *bureau des constatations* that sees Marie's so-called miraculous healing verified.

The Marian Cult and the Female Body

The fact that the novel relies on Pierre's memories of these doctor–patient encounters in order to recount them, as well as the focus on Beauclair's physical examination of Marie, results in this passage marginalizing Marie's own voice

[23] Zola, *Lourdes*, pp. 67–8.
[24] Ibid., p. 68.
[25] Jean-Martin Charcot, *La Foi qui guérit* (Paris: Félix Alcan, 1897), p. 4.
[26] Ibid., p. 5.
[27] Zola, *Lourdes*, p. 68.

and illness experience. The centrality of the body to Marie's medical encounters, and the authority of the doctor over it, necessitates a discussion of the cultural and medical discourses that surrounded the female body in the late nineteenth century: namely the cult of female virginity and corporeal purity. Although *Lourdes* was published before what Henri Mitterand terms the third or even fourth incarnation of Zola, the novel has much in common with its successors, particularly in terms of sharing their natalist ideology. In this vein, Carol Mossman characterizes Zola's 1899 novel *Fécondité* as the author's 'authoritarian hymn to fertility' insofar as it examines obstacles to reproduction, national renewal, and colonial domination.[28] These motifs are present in a number of Zola's novels, often as concluding images: *La Faute de l'abbé Mouret* ends with the birth of a calf to a cow; *Le Docteur Pascal* concludes with an image of Pascal's child being breastfed by its mother.[29] For its part, *Lourdes* is critical of Catholicism in the late nineteenth-century since it promoted a sterile model of femininity for young women.[30] The following section understands *Lourdes* as expounding this natalist theory of female hysteria against the backdrop of the Marian cult's revival at the end of the nineteenth century. This cultural, religious, and medical discourse defines what is at stake in the doctor–patient encounters we see towards the end of the novel.

Marie's physical invalidism is manifested primarily through her inability to walk. In his depiction of Marie's disability, Zola builds on a relatively common analogy between female hysteria (manifested as lower-leg paralysis) and a rejection of maternity. Lucien Israel argues that hysterical paralysis of the legs was an attempted escape from the biological functions expected of the mature female body: '[Les] paralysies [...] constituent, comme tout symptôme hystérique, une représentation, la représentation d'un corps imaginaire auquel manquerait peut-être une fonction par rapport au corps réel, mais on pourrait se demander aussi s'il ne s'agit pas d'un corps débarrassé de certaines fonctions ou activités imposés au corps réel' ['Paralysis constitutes, like any hysterical symptom, a representation, the representation of an imaginary body which would perhaps lack a function in relation to the real body, but one might also wonder whether if it is not about a body freed from certain functions or activities imposed on the real body'].[31] Michael Finn similarly characterizes Rachilde's own lower-limb paralysis as an escape from reproductive heteronormativity by staging 'an acceptance

[28] Carol A. Mossman, *Politics and Narratives of Birth: Gynocolonization from Rousseau to Zola* (Cambridge; New York : Cambridge University Press, 1993), p. 201.

[29] Émile Zola, *La Faute de l'abbé Mouret*, ed. by Colette Becker (Paris: Flammarion, 1999), p. 383; Émile Zola, *Le Docteur Pascal* ed. by Henri Mitterand (Paris: Gallimard, 2017), p. 429.

[30] Henri Mitterand, 'Le Quatrième Zola', *OEuvres et critiques*, 16.2 (1991), 85–98. For a shift in Zola's approach to science after the completion of *Les Rougon-Macquart*, see Michel Gosme, 'Le Nouveau statut de la science dans *Les Trois Villes*', *Cahiers naturalistes*, 74 (2000), 223–36.

[31] Lucien Israël, *L'Hystérique, le sexe et le médecin* (Paris: Masson, 2001), p. 25.

and a performance' of hysteria.[32] The association between paralysis and hysteria was thus a relatively well-established trope in *fin-de-siècle* French literature and Beauclair's location of the cause of Marie's condition in her ovaries points towards a similarly psycho-sexual cause of her paralysis. Indeed, Marie's paralysis is neither wholly invented nor wholly real: it is the embodied memory of the physical trauma sustained through a horse-riding accident, which also coincided with the emotional trauma of puberty: 'une chute de cheval qu'elle avait faite, à treize ans, au moment où elle allait devenir femme' ['a fall from a horse at the age of thirteen, just as she was about to become a woman'].[33] After the accident, Marie became locked in a fragile, childlike body: 'elle était si amaigrie, qu'elle en semblait diminuée, retournée à la taille d'une enfant' ['she was so emaciated that she seemed diminished, returned to the size of a child'].[34] Her childishness equates to her being frozen in a moment in which she is unable to conceive, and thus she is not fully a woman: towards the end of the novel she is described as 'cette enfantine délicieuse, petite fille à vingt-trois ans, restée toujours à la minute où un accident l'avait frappée dans son sexe, l'attardant, l'empêchant d'être femme' ['this delightful child, a little girl aged twenty-three, who always remained at the minute an accident had struck her in her sex, delaying her, preventing her from becoming a woman'].[35] I tackle the potential of seeing Marie's paralysis as an urform of psychosomatic illness in this chapter's final section, but now I wish to focus on how Marie's body is itself configured via the doctor–patient relationship where competing discourses of feminine corporeality in the late nineteenth-century are played out.

Marie's childlike frame recalls what historians have characterized as Catholic mysticism's rejection of maternal reproduction, such as through anorexia and amenorrhea (the cessation of menstruation that can accompany anorexia). Rudolph Bell, for example, compares the lives of the female saints to modern-day discourse surrounding the assumption of a childlike body in sufferers of eating disorders.[36] Although *Lourdes* does not go so far as to directly evoke anorexia, Marie nevertheless remains physically undeveloped and childlike. Her inability to mature into a woman is grounded in her willing ignorance of sexual knowledge: 'On ne peut demander encore ni aux enfants ni aux femmes l'héroïsme amer de la raison' ['The bitter heroism of reason cannot be asked of neither children nor women'].[37] Elsewhere in *Les Rougon-Macquart*, Zola compares infantilization to emasculation, itself understood as a comparable state of ignorance. In *La Faute de*

[32] Michael R. Finn, 'Doctors, Malady, and Creativity in Rachilde', *Nineteenth-Century French Studies*, 34.1–2 (2005), p. 123.

[33] Zola, *Lourdes*, p. 54.

[34] Ibid., p. 64.

[35] Ibid., p. 393.

[36] Rudolph M. Bell, *Holy Anorexia* (Chicago, IL; London: University of Chicago Press, 1985). See also Joan Jacobs Brumberg, *Fasting Girls: The History of Anorexia Nervosa* (New York: Vintage, 2000).

[37] Zola, *Lourdes*, p. 549.

l'abbé Mouret, Serge's rejection of science and turn towards Catholicism is seen as a return to childishness: 'Il ne savait plus, il n'était plus qu'une candeur, qu'une enfance ramenée aux balbutiements du catéchisme' ['He didn't know anymore; he was nothing but candour, a childhood brought back to the beginnings of the catechism'].[38] In *Lourdes*, Zola criticizes the Church for inculcating a hysterical cult of virginity, propagated through an extended attachment to a childlike body. The novel suggests that the phenomenon of Lourdes, including its cures, is only 'un accident explicable' ['an explainable accident'] attributable to 'l'antique forme du catholicisme' ['the old form of Catholicism'].[39] This idea of an antiquated form of Catholicism refers to the revival of the medieval Marian cult in the nineteenth century, to which Marie's name is a clear reference. The Immaculate Conception became dogma in 1854, coinciding with a series of apparitions: the Médaille miraculeuse in Paris in 1830, Notre-Dame de la Salette in 1846, and Lourdes in 1858.[40] Barbara Corrado Pope outlines how, in the face of growing secularization thanks to the development of modern science, the Marian cult became more militant in order to counter a decline in religious deference.[41] The growth of the Marian cult coincided with the concerted effort on the part of medical, religious, and legal authorities to define and confine the feminine body in the nineteenth century and the revival of the Marian cult was central to this trend. The nineteenth century was thus witness to 'a concerted effort to codify women's behaviour in imitation of the Virgin, who became the keystone in the education of girls and the role model for women at all stages of their lives'.[42] Underpinned by Zola's own belief in natalism, *Lourdes* criticizes how the Marian cult revival made sex taboo and illustrates the extent to which Marie's reaction to her own puberty perpetuates the hysterical paralysis that prevents her from maturing into a sexually reproductive woman that conformed to conventional ideas about responsible republican citizens. *Lourdes* shows the influence of the Virgin Mary as all-encompassing, providing the vocabulary through which girls such as Marie would interpret their lives.

Marie is presented as one in a long line of devout hysterical women at Lourdes, with the novel characterizing Bernadette as the paradigmatic case. The structure of *Lourdes* is instructive here, since the novel's five sections, corresponding to the five days of the pilgrimage, are each punctuated by an episode from Bernadette's

[38] Zola, *La Faute de l'abbé Mouret*, p. 135.

[39] Zola, *Lourdes*, p. 570.

[40] For the history of the apparitions, and their impact on France in the nineteenth century, see Philippe Boutry, 'Marie, la grande consolatrice de la France au XIXème siècle', *L'Histoire*, 50 (1982), 31–9. For the apparations at Lourdes, see Yves Chiron, *Enquête sur les miracles de Lourdes* (Paris: Perrin, 2008).

[41] Barbara Corrado Pope, 'Immaculate and Powerful: The Marian Revival in the Nineteenth Century', in *Immaculate and Powerful: The Female in Sacred and Social Reality*, ed. by Clarissa W. Atkinson, Constance H. Buchanan, and Margaret R. Miles (Wellingborough: Crucible, 1987), pp. 176–7.

[42] Patricia A. McEachern, '"La Vierge et La Bête": Marian Iconographies and Bestial Effigies in Nineteenth-Century French Narratives', *Nineteenth-Century French Studies*, 31.1/2 (2002), 111–22 (p. 113).

life and her experience with the Marian apparition. Kathleen Ann Comfort points out that the novel's recounting of Bernadette's tragic demise reflects Marie's illness experience, suggesting the extent to which Marie has absorbed Catholic doctrine into her own experience of illness.[43] During Bernadette's hallucinations, she shouts, 'Va-t'en, va-t'en Satan! Laisse-moi mourir stérile!' ['Get out, get out, Satan! Let me die barren!'].[44] Through her cries, Bernadette reveals the extent to which she equates fertility and maternity with the devil, an association derived from the Church's sanctioning of the Immaculate Conception and, instead, clings onto sterility. Like Bernadette, Marie's childlike nature is made more permanent by her absorption of Catholicism's cult of virginity: she believes that she must have the unspotted soul of a child to guarantee her miraculous cure: 'Père, je sens que je guérirais, si j'avais dix ans, si j'avais l'âme toute blanche d'une petite fille' ['Father, I feel that I would recover if I was ten years old, if I had the unspotted soul of a little girl'].[45] Her pursuit of virginity is reflected in her vow to the Virgin Mary after her cure. Confiding in Pierre, she confesses that:

> Pendant la nuit d'amour, vous savez, la nuit d'extase brûlante que j'ai passé devant la Grotte, je me suis engagée par un vœu, j'ai promis à la Sainte Vierge de lui faire le don de ma virginité, si elle me guérissait [...]. Elle m'a guérie, et jamais, vous entendez, Pierre! Jamais je n'épouserai personne![46]
>
> During that night of love, you know, the night of burning ecstasy that I spent in front of the Grotto, I made a vow: I promised the Blessed Virgin to give her the gift of my virginity if she healed me [...]. She healed me and never, you hear, Pierre! Never will I marry anyone!

Marie here prizes virginity above all else, and therefore it seems right to her that a physical cure would come at the cost of her maternal function. Like a nun, she renounces carnal sexuality and sexual reproduction in favour of holy devotion.

An important observation here is the extent to which Marie's paralysis, and the Marian cult more broadly, can alternatively be understood as tool for self-liberation and defiance. The critical precedent for this interpretation is found in medieval history: Monica Furlong points out how, for nuns during the Middle Ages, mysticism provided a route towards female self-possession, self-knowledge, and rebellion against the Church.[47] Thompson argues that Marie's sense of *pudeur* ['modesty'] effectively repels the doctor's, and the novel's, penetrating medical

[43] Kathleen Ann Comfort, 'Divine Images of Hysteria in Emile Zola's *Lourdes*', *Nineteenth-Century French Studies*, 30.3/4 (2002), 329–45.

[44] Zola, *Lourdes*, p. 568.

[45] Ibid., p. 97.

[46] Ibid., p. 551.

[47] Monica Furlong, *Visions and Longings: An Anthology of Women Mystics* (London: Mowbray, 1996), pp. vii–viii.

gaze.[48] Marie's thinness can thus be understood as a way to reject sexual maturity and the labours of child-bearing, and her politicized body explains Pierre's and the narrator's almost obsessive interest in her. This appropriation of the virginity cult acts as a way for women to rebel against the heteronormative and reproductive roles of wife and mother conventionally accorded to women by the Church. Although *Lourdes* revolves around Marie and her illness, it is striking that the novel's voices of authority belong to male characters who embody either religious or scientific authority or, in the case of Pierre, the authority of a cynic. Potential female authority figures, such as Marie as an authority on her own body or the nuns who perform most of the day-to-day patient care, are marginalized by the text.

Reflecting on the medical scenes already described, we can see that Marie's hysterical paralysis, and her encounter with Beauclair, take place against this backdrop of religious discourse that prized female sexual purity. In contrast to this discursive landscape, *Lourdes* depicts medicine as appearing on the side of fertile maternity and sexual reproduction. Beauclair illustrates that Marie's physical healing will be tantamount to an embrace of heteronormative and sexually reproductive models of femininity:

> Beauclair avait ajouté que Marie serait femme enfin, que le sang de la maternité jaillirait, dans ce sursaut d'hosanna, ce réveil d'un corps resté enfant, attardé et brisé par un si long rêve de souffrance, tout d'un coup rendu à une santé éclatante, les yeux vivants, la face radieuse.[49]

> Beauclair added that Marie would be a woman at last, that the blood of maternity would flow, in this burst of hosanna, this awakening of a body that had remained that of a child, delayed and broken by such a long dream of suffering, suddenly given to a dazzling health, lively eyes, a radiant face.

Beauclair, whose name evokes clear-sightedness and enlightenment ('clair' ['clear']), here takes on a clairvoyant role, continuing Zola's convention of using medical characters, through their diagnosis of certain pathologies, to foretell the course the narrative the novel in question will take.[50] Indeed, Beauclair predicts how Marie will experience her cure: 'en coup de foudre, dans un réveil, une exaltation de tout l'être, tandis que le mal, ce mauvais poids diabolique qui étouffait la jeune fille, remonterait une dernière fois et s'échapperait, comme s'il lui sortait par la bouche' ['very suddenly, in an awakening, an exaltation of the whole being, while the illness, this bad, evil weight which choked the young girl, would

[48] Thompson, *Taboo*, pp. 55–7.
[49] Zola, *Lourdes*, p. 398.
[50] Peter Cryle, 'Foretelling Pathology: The Poetics of Prognosis', *French Cultural Studies*, 17.1 (2006), 107–22.

rise one last time and escape, as if it came out of her mouth'].[51] Moreover, this passage's 'prescription' of sexual reproduction as the ultimate cure for Marie borders on the myth of therapeutic rape as a cure for sexually transgressive women in the nineteenth century.[52] Here, *Lourdes* comes close to what Matlock describes as the framing in *Madame Bovary* of reproductive sex as a 'cure' for female hysteria, thereby recuperating the female hysteric's transgressive body into paradigms of heterosexual desire and production. She thus argues that Emma Bovary's doctors 'would not have granted [her] a divorce; nor would they have left her to books and adulterous affairs. Rather they would have demanded that Charles Bovary find a way to convince her to like sex with him'.[53]

Lourdes thus imagines an idealized doctor–patient encounter in which, firstly, the doctor understands hysterical paralysis to be fuelled by religious discourse revolving around the Marian cult, and, secondly, removes this belief as an obstacle to the patient's maternal fulfilment. This conception of medicine builds on the idealized doctor–patient relationship discussed in Chapter One. However, the novel's ostensible belief in medicine's ability to heal Marie's hysteria, by embracing sexually reproductive relations, does not equate to the patient's liberation. Instead, Marie's rejection of sexual relations through her hysterical paralysis could be understood as a form of defiance against heteronormativity, and that medicine's attempt to 'heal' her is in fact an attempt to force her body to conform to expectations of sexual reproduction. The novel achieves this by inverting the common insinuation that doctors threatened their female patient's sexual purity. Fear of transgressive sexual activity haunted the beginnings of Charcot's hysteria medicine: in Mesmer's era, the potential eroticism of the physical intimacy between magnetizer and patient was the subject of a generalized cultural anxiety. For example, the Faculty of Medicine's secret report on Mesmerism pays attention to the fact that, during the medical encounter,

> La proximité devient la plus grande possible, le visage touche presque le visage, les haleines se respirent, toutes les impressions physiques se partagent instantanément, et l'attraction réciproque des sexes doit agir dans toute sa force; il n'est pas extraordinaire que les sens s'allument. L'imagination, qui agit en même temps, répand un certain désordre dans toute la machine; elle suspend le jugement, elle écarte l'attention; les femmes ne peuvent se rendre compte de ce qu'elles éprouvent, elles ignorent l'état où elles sont.[54]

[51] Zola, *Lourdes*, p. 68.

[52] Bram Dijkstra, *Idols of Perversity: Fantasies of Feminine Evil in Fin-de-Siècle Culture* (New York: Oxford University Press, 1988), pp. 64–82.

[53] See Matlock, *Scenes of Seduction*, p. 157.

[54] Alexandre Bertrand, 'Rapport secret sur le magnétisme, par Bailly et ses collègues', in *Du magnétisme animal en France* (Paris: J. Baillère, 1826), p. 513.

> The proximity becomes as great as possible, one face almost touches another, the two breaths intermingle, all physical sensations are shared instantaneously, and the reciprocal attraction of the sexes must act in all its force. It is not unusual for the senses to become aroused; the imagination, which acts at the same time, spreads a certain disorder throughout the body, it suspends judgement, it distracts attention; women can't comprehend what they are feeling; they do not know the state they are in.

In this passage, the encounter between Mesmerist and patient is clearly framed in terms of physical connection and sexual threat. Indeed, Lindsay Wilson describes how Mesmerism's deliberate incitation of convulsions provoked a pamphlet war that rallied to the cause of exposing Mesmerism as a threat to sexual and moral propriety.[55] But by the time of *Lourdes*, the greatest threat to sexual and reproductive mores are seen as emanating from the Church's ostensible indoctrination of young girls into the Marian cult. In the novel, the medical encounter appears as the potential cure for the Church's virginal cult, thereby inverting medical and religious authority. Whereas scholars such as Matlock and Beizer have characterized the doctor as deliberately harming his patients for the sake of their sexual correction; in *Lourdes* the Church is characterized as manipulating and injuring young women. In the medical encounter, then, doctors such as Beauclair protect these female patients through a quasi-Mesmerist embrace of the mysterious way in which the body and mind are connected in hysteria. Zola presents the doctor–patient encounter as the antidote to the relationship cultivated between Church and young *dévotes* that precluded the sexual reproduction defined by natalism to be essential to a young woman's social worth and thus physical health. The doctor–patient encounter thus facilitates the understanding and cure of Marie by resisting the Church's ideology of sexual purity. Conversely, Marie's thinness can, at the same time, be understood as a way in which the character rejects sexual maturity and the labours of childbearing. Women's appropriation of the virginity cult allows them to rebel against the heteronormative and reproductive roles of wife and mother conventionally accorded to women by the Church. Although *Lourdes* revolves around Marie and her illness, it is striking that the novel's voices of authority belong to male characters who embody either religious or scientific authority or, in the case of Pierre, doubt and cynicism. The novel's focus on the dichotomy between religion and science privileges male characters at the expense of female characters, since these female voices are lost in the novel's lengthy debates about the relative virtues

[55] Lindsay B. Wilson, *Women and Medicine in the French Enlightenment: The Debate over 'maladies des femmes'* (Baltimore, MD; London: Johns Hopkins University Press, 1993), pp. 110–24.

of religion and science, recounted in free indirect discourse focalized through Pierre.[56]

Of Germs and Miracles

The debate between feminine sexual reproductivity and the cult of virginity is echoed by another late-nineteenth-century battleground: the scientific interest in germ theory on the one hand, and the Church's renewed emphasis on miracles on the other. In the middle of the nineteenth century, Louis Pasteur's discovery of microbes threatened to undermine the epistemological foundation on which the doctor–patient relationship and encounter had previously been based. As Bruno Latour states: 'Le biologiste ou le physiologiste [...] s'intéressent à des acteurs *internes* parfois microscopiques parfois fonctionnels [...]. Ils parlent d'organe, de fonction glycogénique du foie, de respiration, de cellules. Voilà un monde immense qui n'interfère [pas] directement [...] avec le 'colloque singulier' des médecins' ['The biologist or physiologist [...] is interested in sometimes microscopic and other times functional *internal* actors [...]. They speak of the organ, the glycogenic function of the liver, respiration, cells. Here is a huge world that does not directly interfere with the "singular colloquium" of doctors'].[57] Like the discourse around sexual reproduction, the battleground of germs and miracles impinged on the doctor–patient relationship. The medical relationship, the 'colloque singulier' between doctors and their patients, was at risk because of the progress of microbiology and laboratory-based science. Latour states that Pasteur's interest in microbes and their relative virulence amounted to an epistemological shift in medicine that subverted the social arrangement of the bedside around which clinical practice had hitherto been organized. With such an agent as microbes, Pasteur and his disciples 'peuvent [...] se rire des catégories avec lesquelles la société du 19e siècle est bâtie' ['can [...] make light of the categories on which nineteenth-century society was built'].[58] One of these categories was the knowledge on which the physician's authority was built: knowledge of the patient and their body.[59] Latour's depiction of a practice-based medicine that was being uprooted by a new, science-based medicine recalls Foucault's own argument that removing the

[56] Julia Przybos describes Pierre as Zola's 'mouthpiece'. See Julia Przybos, 'Zola's Utopias', in *The Cambridge Companion to Émile Zola*, ed. by Brian Nelson (Cambridge: Cambridge University Press, 2007), pp. 169–87 (p. 175).

[57] Bruno Latour, *Les Microbes: guerre et paix; suivi de, Irréductions* (Paris: A. M. Métailié, 1984), p. 116, original emphasis. For a comprehensive overview of this phenomenon, see Laura Otis, *Membranes: Metaphors of Invasion in Nineteenth-Century Literature, Science, and Politics* (Baltimore, MD; London: Johns Hopkins University Press, 1999).

[58] Latour, *Les Microbes*, p. 116.

[59] Ibid., p. 116.

patient's individuality from medical enquiry at the turn of the nineteenth century was the first move towards the modernization of medicine.[60] The process of scientization, identified by Foucault as beginning in the early nineteenth century and ostensibly completed by the 1850s, appears in the work of contemporary doctors. To give only one example, in his work on the bacillus responsible for the bubonic plague, the Swiss doctor Alexandre Yersin erases the patient from his work, referring exclusively to *la maladie* ['the disease'] rather than *le malade* ['the sick person'], *le moribond* ['the dying person'], or *le convalescent* ['the convalescing person'] throughout his description of bubonic plague.[61]

Despite this tendency, in *Lourdes* we see a re-affirmation of the doctor–patient relationship's centrality to medicine because of its ability to capture what is invisible and to provide pathways to healing through an understanding of the invisible. According to Latour, the discovery of microbes meant that society, and in particular the medical community, was required to make room for the invisible: 'À composer la société avec seulement des liens sociaux en omettant les invisibles, on aboutit à une corruption générale, à une déviation perverse des bonnes volontés humaines. Pour agir efficacement d'homme à homme [...] il faut "faire place" aux microbes' ['To compose society with only social bonds while omitting the invisible ones, there would be a general corruption, a perverse deviation of human good will. In order to act effectively from man to man [...] we must "make room" for microbes'].[62] This 'making room for the invisible' is perceptible in *fin-de-siècle* literature's interest in the unknown and the unknowable. For example, in Maupassant's *Le Horla* the physical atmosphere is characterized as containing mysterious invisible elements: 'D'où viennent ces influences mystérieuses qui changent en découragement notre bonheur et notre confiance en détresse. On dirait que l'air, l'air invisible est plein d'inconnaissables Puissances, dont nous subissons les voisinages mystérieux' ['Where do these mysterious influences come from that turn our happiness into despondency and our confidence into distress? It seems that the air, the invisible air, is full of unknowable powers, whose mysterious parts we are subjected to'].[63] Not only did the development of this microscopic vision emphasize what was previously unseeable or unknowable, it did not undermine the doctor–patient relationship as a nexus of knowledge. In fact, it strengthened this traditional form of medicine: Latour argues that 'La dérive ou le déplacement pastorien [...] offre aux médecins à partir de 1894 un moyen de continuer leur métier traditionnel d'hommes qui soignent, mais avec une efficacité *renforcée* par le pastorisme' ['The change or Pastorian displacement [...] offered doctors, from 1894, a means of continuing their traditional profession of men who care [for

60 Foucault, *Naissance de la clinique*, p. 26.
61 Alexandre Yersin, 'La Peste bubonique à Hong Kong', *Annales de l'Institut Pasteur*, 8 (1894), 662–7.
62 Latour, *Les Microbes*, pp. 42–3.
63 Guy de Maupassant, *Le Horla*, ed. by André Fermigier (Paris: Gallimard, 2009), p. 37.

patients], but with an efficiency reinforced by Pastorism'].[64] *Lourdes* in fact reinforces the importance of the doctor–patient relationship to health, but in so doing reconfigures the foundations on which it is constructed.

Holy water is of course central to the cult at Lourdes, but Pasteur's microbiology gave water a renewed importance in scientific discourse. On the one hand, water could eradicate harmful germs; but, on the other hand, it could also carry them. The eradication of germs was characterized as an important moral endeavour, as according to an 1896 pamphlet on public hygiene, 'Le microbe, voilà l'ennemi' ['Germs are the enemy'].[65] This was particularly so given the virulence of water-borne infectious diseases such as typhoid and cholera, described in Zola's *La Faute de l'abbé Mouret* and Sand's *Lélia* respectively. Laura Otis thus observes the combative vocabulary that was used to articulate the new germ theory and its application to public health, notably through the evocation of barriers, frontiers, and battlegrounds.[66] Indeed, regular cleansing with water became more closely and more rigorously associated with scientific needs: Bachelard observes that 'se purifier n'est pas purement et simplement se nettoyer. Et rien n'autorise à parler d'un besoin de propreté comme d'un besoin primitif, que l'homme reconnaîtrait dans sa sagesse native' ['To purify oneself is not purely and simply to clean oneself. And there is nothing that allows us to describe cleanliness as a primitive need, which man would recognize in his native wisdom'].[67] Water, previously associated with Christian rites such as baptism, thus became secularized thanks to Pasteur's advances in microbiology which observed and objectified its properties.[68] In *Lourdes*, the Grotto's waters are characterized through the new discourse of germs, and Zola's use of the new vocabulary of microbiology contributes to his framing of the novel's final doctor–patient encounter. The development of microbiology revealed that water could also be the source of illness and disease and that its purity could not be determined by eye. The safety of water could only be understood by chemical analysis: telling the difference between pure and impure, and how both are defined, becomes a veritable crisis in the novel and one that the doctor–patient relationship attempts to solve.

Concurrently with the revolution in microbiology, the revival of the Marian cult also drew on water to express the new dogma of the Immaculate Conception. The Church used metaphors of water to reinforce its message of feminine purity. Jean Pierrot draws attention to the *fin-de-siècle* interest in the metaphorical potential of water: water is intrinsically capable of expressing the fluidity of

[64] Latour, *Les Microbes*, p. 127.

[65] Cited by Georges Vigarello, in Georges Vigarello, *Histoire des pratiques de santé: le sain et le malsain depuis le Moyen Âge* (Paris: Points, 2016), p. 254.

[66] Otis, *Membranes*, pp. 3–34.

[67] Gaston Bachelard, *L'Eau et les rêves: essai sur l'imagination de la matière* (Paris: J. Corti, 1963), p. 191.

[68] Jean-Pierre Goubert, *La Conquête de l'eau: l'avènement de la santé à l'âge industriel* (Paris: R. Laffont, 1986).

the imaginary realm since it is 'changeante, évanescente, subtile' ['changeable, evanescent, subtle'].[69] These qualities lead Pierrot to argue that water is an innately malleable material for writers: 'Sa signification affective et imaginaire se modifie considérablement [...] selon qu'il s'agit d'une eau courante ou au contraire immobile et dormante, d'eau transparente ou obscure' ['Its affective and imaginary meaning changes considerably [...] depending on whether it is running water or, on the contrary, if it is still and dormant, transparent or dark'].[70] These qualities underpin the Church's obsession with the healing powers of the Lourdes waters: embodying the idealized femininity of the Virgin Mary, the waters at Lourdes are considered to be pure and unblemished. Like the Virgin, they were considered invested with miraculous powers.

On the one hand, the novel presents the pilgrims as defining the waters' supposed purity as evidence of its holiness; on the other hand, the narration maintains that 'purity' should only pertain to hygienic cleanliness, which it believes to be thoroughly lacking at Lourdes. Building on this polarization, Zola's *Lourdes* demonstrates the extent to which water became a battleground between the so-called competing interests of science, who associated water with germ theory and hygiene, and religion, who prized certain waters for their ability to perform miracles. *Lourdes* traces how, according to Bachelard, unnatural and misplaced faith in the cleansing power of dirty waters becomes a metaphor for the circulation of disease contrary to modern scientific practice. The waters are characterized as a 'bouillon terrible' ['horrible broth'] of germs and disease: 'Quelle saleté, quelle bouillon de microbes!... La manie, la fureur de précautions antiseptiques où nous sommes, reçoit là un fameux soufflet. Comment se fait-il qu'une même peste n'emporte pas tous ces malades? Les adversaires de la théorie microbienne doivent bien rire' ['What filth, what a broth of germs...! The mania, the fury of hygiene precautions in which we find ourselves, receives a heavy blow. How is it that one plague does not get rid of all the ill people? The opponents of germ theory must be having a good laugh'].[71] The novel attributes the state of the waters to the priests' neglect of basic hygiene, which they deprioritize in favour of preserving the water's supposed healing powers: 'l'eau [...] n'était guère engageante; car, de crainte que le débit de la source ne pût suffire, les pères de la Grotte ne faisaient alors changer l'eau des baignoires que deux fois par jour' ['The water [...] was hardly inviting because, for fear that the amount produced by the source would not be enough, the Grotto priests only changed the water in the bathtubs twice a day'].[72] The Grotto's healing waters become a soup of germs in which various illnesses mingle and threaten the life of all those willing to submerge themselves in its water:

[69] Jean Pierrot, *L'Imaginaire décadent (1880–1900)* (Mont-Saint-Aignan: Publications des universités de Rouen et du Havre, 2007), p. 258.
[70] Ibid.
[71] Zola, *Lourdes*, p. 212.
[72] Ibid., p. 192.

'Il s'y rencontrait de tout, des filets de sang, des débris de peau, des croûtes, des morceaux de charpie et de bandage, un affreux consommé de tous les maux, de toutes les plaies, de toutes les pourritures' ['Everything was in there, streaks of blood, flakes of skin, scabs, pieces of shredded cloth and bandages, an awful soup of all the ailments, all the wounds, of all the rot'].[73]

The priests' neglect of hygiene metonymically represents Catholicism's prioritizing of the invisible, the divine purity of the water by refusing to change it, over the visible signs of its contamination. Miracles make visible the otherwise invisible work of a divine being: a convincing miracle 'peuplait l'invisible' ['populated the invisible'] and gives the pilgrims hope that they will also be cured since the miracles 'montrait à chaque malade son ange gardien derrière lui, prêt à l'assister, sur un ordre du Ciel' ['showed each sick person the guardian angel standing behind him, ready to assist by order of Heaven'].[74] Although Zola's novel condemns religious faith, it does not exclude the importance of scientific faith which, in accordance with the new Pastorian medicine, likewise required faith in what was invisible, but whose existence could be proved through chemical analysis: 'Il semblait que ce fût une véritable culture des germes empoisonneurs, une essence des contagions les plus redoutables, et le miracle devait être que l'on ressortît vivant de cette boue humaine' ['It seemed to be a veritable culture of poisonous germs, a variety of the most formidable contagions, and the miracle was surely that anyone emerged alive from that human filth'].[75] The stench of the Grotto's waters contrasts with the heavenly floral scents associated with the Virgin. In *Les Foules de Lourdes*, Huysmans insists on the putrefaction of the waters by patients. For example, their shirts are 'maculée[s], par endroit, de gomme-gutte et de sang frais, empesée, à d'autres, par des taches d'humeur sèche qui la font ressembler à du sparadrap' ['smeared with dried bile and blood, and there were dry patches that made it look like a bandage'].[76]

Moreover, the Grotto's waters are described in *Lourdes* as not only a fetid stew of germs and disease but additionally frigidly cold. Monsieur Sabathier is particularly traumatized by his experience in the Grotto: 'L'eau froide le terrifiait. Il racontait encore que, la première fois, il avait éprouvé un saisissement si atroce, qu'il s'était juré de ne recommencer jamais. À l'entendre, il n'y avait pas de pire torture' ['The cold water terrified him. He was still telling the story of how, the first time, he had felt such a terrible shock he had promised himself never to do it again. To hear him tell it, there could be no worse torture'].[77] As Jacques Noiray observes, coolness in *Lourdes* is associated with, on the one hand, the supposedly miraculous waters but, on the other hand, life-giving freshness. This contrast is best

[73] Ibid., pp. 192–3.
[74] Ibid., p. 103.
[75] Ibid., p. 193.
[76] Joris-Karl Huysmans, *Les Foules de Lourdes* (Paris: Stock, 1906), p. 63.
[77] Zola, *Lourdes*, p. 192.

seen in the omnipresence of the river Gave in the novel, which Zola characterizes as life-giving: the 'grand ciel de lumière et de joie où montait la fraîcheur du Gave' ['great sky of light and joy where the freshness of the Gave came from'], and particularly the river's 'eaux limpides, vertes et bleues' ['blue-green transparent waters'] and the lush surrounding landscape.[78] Given the Church's insistent on abstinence and female sexual purity, it does not seem too much of a stretch to associate the coldness of the Grotto's waters with sexual frigidity and the failure of reproduction.

This characterization of the waters as freezing cold and contaminated contrasts with how knowledge is conceived in the novel. In contrast to the pools of ignorance in the Grotto, the free-flowing river Gave incarnates truth: 'La vérité bouillonnait, débordait, en un tel flot irrésistible' ['Truth was bubbling, overflowing, in such an uncontrollable stream'].[79] Water is thus a mobile symbol in the novel, representing both *vérité* in its free-flowing state as well as the Church's scientific ignorance and Marie's hysterical frigidity through the polluted, freezing waters of the Grotto. The revolution in microbiology thus heralded a confrontation between two conceptions of water. Scientific writers saw water as a resource which required sterilization to combat invisible, but material, microbes; yet, at the same time, Catholics understood it as a sacrament whose invisible qualities rendered it holy. *Lourdes* confronts the intersection between the development of microbiological science, seen as an intellectually fertile ground, on the one hand, and the stagnant and frigid Marian cult's aquatic metaphors, on the other. In the final section of this chapter, I discuss in more detail how the novel reconfigures the doctor–patient relationship to suggest that this binary between science and faith is illusory.

These competing understandings of water converge in the novel converge at the site of the doctor–patient relationship. Beauclair's insistence that the pilgrimage to Lourdes will heal Marie, or rather allow her to heal herself, is instructive. For him, despite the waters' health risks, the spiritual experience of taking the waters will allow Marie to overcome both the mental and physical aspects of her disability. Returning to the novel's initial framing device thus allows the reader an early glimpse into the redemptive doctor–patient relationship that the rest of the novel will attempt to formulate.

The filthiness of the Grotto's water elicits both repulsion and fear and, like the novel's depiction of hysteria in the doctor–patient relationship, organizes these responses around the female body. Zola uses Lourdes's waters to create a contrast between two conceptions of femininity, ironically underpinned by their mutual transgression from heterosexual reproduction. As we have already seen, Marie and

[78] Ibid., p. 172.
[79] Ibid., p. 60.

Bernadette embody the Church's conception of virginal sterility as outlined previously. But Élise Rouquet, a woman suffering from lupus as well as a facial wound, embodies the antithetical features of vice and corrupted sexuality, since she is the novel's central incarnation of femininity turned into monstrosity by the repulsive effects of disease.[80] The ulceration of her facial scar is dramatically revealed in its entire horrifying state:

> Enfin, le fichu tomba, et Marie eut un frisson d'horreur. C'était un lupus, qui avait envahi le nez et la bouche, peu à peu grandi là, une ulcération lente s'étalant sans cesse sous les croûtes, dévorant les muqueuses. La tête allongée en museau de chien, avec ses cheveux rudes et ses gros yeux ronds, était devenue affreuse. Maintenant, les cartilages du nez se trouvaient presque mangés, la bouche s'était rétractée, tirée à gauche par l'enflure de la lèvre supérieure, pareille à une fente oblique, immonde et sans forme. Une sueur de sang, mêlée à du pus, coulait de l'énorme plaie livide.[81]

> Finally, the scarf fell off, and Marie experienced a chill of terror. It was a lupus which had invaded her nose and mouth, had grown there little by little, a slow ulceration spreading incessantly underneath the scabs, devouring her mucous membranes. Her head, stretched out like a dog's muzzle, with her coarse hair and big round eyes, had become hideous. Now the nose's cartilage was almost eaten away, the mouth had sunken in and was pulled to the left by the swelling in the upper lip, which was like a slanted slit, filthy and shapeless. Blood mixed with pus oozed from the huge, livid sore.

In this passage, the reader encounters abject bodily fluids denoting the corporeality of the female body, and the feeling of terror produced on the onlooker echoes my discussion of the exploitation of abject symptoms for metaphorical potential in Stendhal's *Lamiel* and Sand's *Lélia*. However, by locating Élise's illness both visibly and prominently (namely on her face), the scar reveals more than it may first appear. As Rothfield reminds us, Laclos's *Les Liaisons dangereuses* is a potentially fruitful intertext for Zola's work.[82] This novel reveals the link between female patient's facial disfigurement and an insinuation as to their supposedly wayward sexual and moral habits. In *Nana*, the eponymous courtesan's face famously becomes scarred with smallpox, and the etymological connection between smallpox, *la petite vérole*, and syphilis, *la grande vérole*, suggests how the former disease was often used to insinuate the latter and thus the venereal occupational hazards of

[80] McEachern, 'La Vierge et La Bête', p. 120.
[81] Zola, *Lourdes*, p. 45.
[82] Rothfield, for example, characterizes the difference between Laclos's and Zola's depiction of disease as coalescing around the development of microscopic sciences around the mid-point of the nineteenth century. See Rothfield, *Vital Signs*, p. 7.

prostitution.[83] The horror experienced at the sight of Élise's wound is only heightened when the filthy reality of the shared water tap in the Grotto is revealed, again made visible thanks to the 'discovery' of microbes:

> [Pierre] fut surtout intéressé par le spectacle d'Élise Rouquet qui, jugeant inutile d'aller aux piscines, pour la plaie affreuse dont sa face était rongée, se contentait, depuis le matin, de se lotionner à la fontaine, toutes les heures. Elle s'agenouillait, écartait le fichu, appliquait longuement sur la plaie un mouchoir qu'elle imbibait, comme une éponge.[84]

> [Pierre] was particularly interested by the spectacle of Élise Rouquet who, since that morning, seeing it as futile to go the pools because of the hideous sore on her face, had been content to lotion herself at the fountain every hour. She would kneel down, push her veil away, and for a long time she would dab the wound with her handkerchief which she soaked [in the waters] like a sponge.

The crowd's mania for the waters is such that they ignore its contamination: 'autour d'[Élise], la foule se ruait dans une telle fièvre, que les gens ne remarquaient plus son visage de monstre, se lavaient et buvaient au canon même où elle mouillait son mouchoir' ['around [Élise], the crowd rushed in such a fever that people no longer noticed her monstrous face, and they washed and drank from the same water in which she soaked her handkerchief'].[85]

The fact of the sexual-symbolic dimension of Élise's facial lupus thus suggests a sexual transgression that wreaks a toll on the woman's body. By foregrounding how sexual behaviour becomes inscribed on the body, and thus becomes indecipherable to others, the body of the alleged prostitute is aligned with that of the hysteric-virgin Marie, whose paralysis is equally a physical manifestation of her own sexual mores. The potential contagion risk of the syphilitic prostitute is a not-too-distant cousin from the trope of the hysteric: Mark Micale insists on the importance of 'hystero-syphilis' that was developed at the end of the century and become a common trope in both literary and medical discourse.[86] Moreover, the pathogenic, and not just nervous, cause and thus potential transmission of mania is highlighted in Zola's 'Ébauche' ['Sketch'] for *La Faute de l'abbé Mouret*: 'Serge est tombé malade d'une fièvre typhoïde affreuse' ['Serge

[83] Bertrand Taithe, *Defeated Flesh: Welfare, Warfare and the Making of Modern France* (Manchester: Manchester University Press, 1999), p. 218. See also Wilson, *The Language of Disease*, pp. 33–5 and 45–6.

[84] Zola, *Lourdes*, p. 190.

[85] Ibid., p. 190.

[86] Mark S. Micale, *The Mind of Modernism: Medicine, Psychology, and the Cultural Arts in Europe and America, 1880–1940* (Stanford, CA: Stanford University Press, 2004), p. 83.

has fallen ill with an awful typhoid fever'].[87] Throughout the novel, Serge's fever progresses from a light and seemingly inconsequential fever to a full-blown religious mania, anticipating *Lourdes*'s speculation about the cause of hysterical diseases.

One of these causes is suggested to be that the hysterical mania for miracles can spread as a form of nervous contagion or mass hysteria, building on the discourse of germ theory illustrated previously. Marie walks for the first time at the height of a frenzied series of chapters detailing the Grotto chapel service on the final day of the official pilgrimage. In the build-up to this event, Zola describes how the priest leads the congregation in a fervent chanting: 'la foule sanglota après lui [...]. Puis, coup sur coup, les appels s'entêtèrent à crier de plus en plus haut la misère exaspérée du monde [...]. C'était du délire' ['The crowd wept after him [...]. Then, one after the other, the calls continued to ring out, louder and louder, the exasperated misery of the people [...]. It was madness'].[88] Throughout this section, Zola refers to the indomitable power of the crowd: the 'poussées inconscientes de la foule' ['the unconscious pushing of the crowd'], the 'mur impénétrable de la foule' ['the impenetrable wall of the crowd'], 'le flot mouvant' ['the moving flow'], and a 'foule sans bornes' ['boundless crowd'].[89] Focalized through Pierre, the narration insists that although the crowd poses little physical danger, it is nonetheless deeply unnerving: 'Pierre n'avait jamais eu une sensation si anxieuse de la foule. Elle était sans menace, d'une innocence et d'une passivité de troupeau; mais il y trouvait un frisson troublant, un souffle particulier qui le bouleversait' ['Pierre had never felt so anxious about crowds. It was not threatening; instead it possessed the innocence and passivity of a herd; but he found in it a disturbing thrill, a particular breath that overwhelmed him'].[90] The characterization of the crowd as a mindless herd underlines the extent to which the crowd is affected and led by the priests.

It is amidst this heightened atmosphere that the miraculous cures begin: 'Tout d'un coup, une paralytique venait de se lever, de marcher vers la Grotte, en tenant sa béquille en l'air' ['All of a sudden, a paralysed woman stood up, walking towards the Grotto, holding her crutch in the air'].[91] Zola insinuates that the crowd's desire to see a miracle encourages them to materialize, which in turn encourages another miracle to occur:

> On guettait les prodiges, on les attendait, avec la certitude qu'ils se produiraient, innombrables, éclatants. Des yeux croyaient les voir, des voix fébriles les signalaient. Encore une autre qui était guérie! Encore une autre! Encore une autre!

[87] Émile Zola, *Les Rougon-Macquart*, ed. by Armand Lanoux and Henri Mitterand, 5 vols (Paris: Gallimard, 1960), I, p. 1693.
[88] Zola, *Lourdes*, p. 387.
[89] Ibid., pp. 388, 390, 391, 393.
[90] Ibid., p. 391.
[91] Ibid., p. 394.

> Une sourde qui entendait, une muette qui parlait, une phtisique qui ressuscitait! Comment, une phtisique? Mais certainement, cela était quotidien! Il n'y avait plus de surprise possible, on aurait constaté sans étonner personne qu'une jambe coupée repoussait.[92]
>
> Prodigies were watched out for, they were waited for, with the certainty that they would occur, innumerable and brilliant. Eyes thought they saw them, feverish voices indicated them. Yet another one had been cured! And another! And another! A deaf woman who could hear again, a mute who could speak again, a tuberculosis patient who had been resuscitated! What, a tuberculosis patient? But, of course, that was an everyday occurrence! It was no longer possible to surprise anyone, it would have been observed without any shock if a severed leg grew back.

This passage traces the crowd's collective desire for miracles ('On guettait les prodiges'), producing eyes that believe they saw them ('Des yeux croyaient les voir'), in turn creating such miraculous events. These miracles are then described as occurring in a chain-reaction, punctuated by the feverish refrain ('Encore une autre'). These miracles are insinuated as becoming increasingly less believable the longer it goes on, suggested by hypophora that instantly responds to any incredulousness, although only through conviction rather than with rational reasoning ('Comment, une phtisique? Mais certainement').

Amidst the crowd's frenetic energy, Marie lifts herself from her wheelchair. As for much of the novel, this moment is focalized through Pierre, who watches her face transform from that of an ill person. The narration recounts that 'Les yeux de la malade, vides encore, [...] son pauvre visage blême' ['The patient's eyes, still empty, [...] her poor pale face'] turns into one filled with light and hope: 'tout d'un coup, lorsque le Saint-Sacrament passa et qu'elle en regarda l'astre flamboyer au soleil, elle eut un éblouissement, elle crut frappé d'un éclair. Ses yeux s'étaient rallumés à cet éclat, ils retrouvaient enfin leur flamme de vie, ils brillaient pareils à des étoiles' ['suddenly, as the Holy Sacrament passed by and she watched its star blaze in the sun, she was dazzled; she thought that she had been struck by lightning. Her eyes rekindled that glow, they finally rediscovered their life spark, they shone like stars'].[93]

Inspired by the proximity of the eucharist, Marie is thrust into health and light for the first time. She slowly begins to lift herself out of her chair and then shouts 'Je suis guérie! Je suis guérie!' ['I'm healed! I'm healed!'].[94]

[92] Ibid., p. 394.
[93] Ibid., p. 402.
[94] Ibid., p. 402.

The depiction of illness and medicine in *Lourdes* is thus extremely broad, ranging from medical to religious discourse, and metaphorically rich, particularly regarding the recurring motif of water. It is this intricate web of metaphors and invisible meaning that Latour argues the nineteenth-century doctor–patient encounter could capture, despite or even because of the revolution in microbiology heralded in by the 1850s. This multi-layered discourse of health and healing at Lourdes in the nineteenth century feeds into the novel's depiction of the medical relationship and encounter and, in turn, necessitates a new formulation of the former.

Towards a New Healing Relationship

Following the scene of mass hysteria in the Grotto, *Lourdes* returns to the doctor–patient encounter and relationship to illustrate the extent to which a belief in the imaginary must be filtered through a trustworthy medical relationship. By demonstrating the extent to which the *bureau des constatations médicales* corrupted the clinical encounter by the doctors' adhesion to Catholic dogma, the novel calls for a new way to understand doctor–patient encounters as primarily vehicles of relief, regardless of the scientific or non-scientific basis of that relief. Whereas Marie's earlier encounter with the *bureau*'s doctors is described as inherently limited by the doctors' predetermined belief in the veracity of miracles, *Lourdes* proposes a surprising alternative model for medicine that not only lacks the limitations that shape Marie's medical experience, but also embraces the breadth of human experience and suffering and responds to it.

After Marie walks unaided from her wheelchair, Pierre tries to focus on how Marie's suffering has been relieved by her cure. But he cannot help remembering Beauclair's diagnosis of 'le simple état d'autosuggestion' ['the simple state of autosuggestion'].[95] Nonetheless, Marie proudly presents herself at the *bureau des constatations médicales* to have her miracle verified by the Lourdes doctors. Marie's examination with a group of medics, rather than a singular doctor, is strongly rem iniscent of the group portrait of Charcot with which this chapter opened. Since Lourdes doctors are sure these doctors could not have misdiagnosed Marie, they conclude that her cure must be miraculous: 'si l'on avait le moindre doute, ces deux certificats suffiraient à convaincre les plus incrédules, car ils sont signés par deux médecins de la Faculté de Paris, dont les noms sont bien connus de tous nos confrères' ['if there was any doubt, these two certificates would be enough to convince even the most incredulous, since they are signed by two doctors from the

[95] Ibid., p. 397.

Faculty of Paris whose names are well known to all our colleagues'].[96] The passage pays particular attention to impression that the Parisan doctors' signatures leaves on the doctors working in Lourdes: 'les signataires avaient la réputation de praticiens honnêtes et habiles' ['the signatories had the reputation of being honest and skilled practitioners'].[97] The medical authority of the signatories, and the fact that Marie's cure cannot be explained by modern science, means that it is quickly certified as miraculous: 'Le cas échappe à la science, voilà tout ce que je constate' ['The case escapes science, that's all that I can say'].[98] Building on the characterization of the Grotto's waters as germ-ridden, morally stagnant, and sexually frigid, Marie's cure emerges as entirely the product of both the physicians' and the patients' steadfast belief in the existence of miracles.

Moreover, Pierre's account of Marie's encounter with the two Parisian doctors points towards the failure of medicine. Pierre remembers the consensus that two Parisian doctors were forced to reach about Marie's diagnosis, and I similarly return to this passage: 'Deux des médecins, [...] l'un croyant à une rupture des ligaments larges, l'autre diagnostiquant une paralysie due à une lésion de la moelle' ['Two of the doctors [...], one believing in a rupture of the broad ligament, the other diagnosing paralysis caused by a lesion of the spinal cord'] but that they nevertheless decide on an explicitly vague diagnosis, 'cette paralysie, avec des accidents, peut-être, du côté des ligaments' ['this paralysis, with perhaps some accident having occurred to her ligaments'].[99] Zola here shows that the doctors failed to undertake any rigorous scientific investigation into the true nature of Marie's original paralysis, instead they merely 'tomber d'accord' ['reached an agreement'] that her ligaments are at fault. Here the verb *tomber* ['to fall'] implies a degree of passivity on their part and the inevitability of their conclusion, rather than the more active alternative *trouver un accord* ['to find an agreement']. The Parisian doctors' omission opens the door to the certification of Marie's miracle: the Parisians' signatures are enough to convince the *bureau* that Marie's paralysis was wholly physical. As in *La Peau de chagrin* and *Lélia*, this scene in the *bureau des constatations médicales* denounces the so-called medical authority of the physicians as bankrupt thanks to their limited understanding of the true workings of illness and health.

Notwithstanding the novel's overt condemnation of this capitulation, the failure of the Parisian and Pyrenean doctor–patient encounters allows *Lourdes*, in its depiction of Beauclair, to imagine a new relationship that prioritizes compassion over adherence to both medical science and to Catholic dogma. Pierre's reluctant endorsement of Marie's cure suggests that science must remain open to the mysterious and the unknown because of the desperation that accompanies human

[96] Ibid., p. 405.
[97] Ibid., p. 405.
[98] Ibid., p. 408.
[99] Ibid., p. 67.

suffering. After Marie's cure Pierre continues to torture himself with the knowledge that Marie's cure has a scientific, rather than divine, explanation, he cannot bring himself to tell her the truth: 'Beauclair le lui avait bien dit que la guérison viendrait en coup de foudre, lorsque, sous l'influence de l'imagination puissamment surexcitée, il se produirait en elle un réveil soudain de la volonté, depuis si longtemps endormie' ['Beauclair had told her that healing would take place very suddenly, at a moment when, under the influence of her over-excited imagination, there would be a sudden awakening of her determination, which had been dormant for so long'].[100] But although this anecdote could explain 'scientifiquement' ['scientifically'] Marie's cure, Pierre does not recount it to the *bureau*, but instead agrees with the doctors, muttering 'C'est vrai, c'est vrai' ['It's true, it's true'].[101] Pierre's desire to see Marie married is not sufficient motivation for him to dispel her belief in her own cure. Instead he feels an 'immense pitié' ['huge pity'] for Marie's suffering.[102] Having witnessed her suffering, Pierre feels morally obliged to prioritize the alleviation of Marie's pain regardless of the origin of that cure: 'il fallait tolérer Lourdes, ainsi qu'on tolère le mensonge qui aide à vivre' ['Lourdes must be tolerated, similarly to how lies are tolerated when they aid living'].[103] In keeping with the novel's general eliding of Pierre with the narrator, the former's personal resolution becomes the novel's general approach to the questions of illness and healing, as well as the doctor–patient relationship and encounter.

While we must avoid the somewhat reductive impulse to diagnose Marie's condition, the connection made by the novel between her emotional trauma and her present physical state resonates with what is now understood to be psychosomatic illness. The field of psychosomatic illness attempts to question the Cartesian dualism between mind and body prevalent in Western society by prioritizing the interconnectedness of these two elements.[104] As Jon Stone observes, prejudice against the term 'psychosomatic' is both entrenched and widespread in twenty-first-century discourse, since it is perceived to be linked with the now-derogatory term 'hysteria' and the off-hand explanation that an illness may be 'all in your head'.[105] Indeed, Suzanne O'Sullivan points out that Charcot's science of hysteria is best understood as a precursor to the twenty-first century field of psychosomatic medicine.[106] Zola's *Lourdes* is no doubt sceptical about Marie's illness: in the final pages of the novel it is suggested that the real cause of Marie's paralysis may

[100] Ibid., pp. 406–7.
[101] Ibid., p. 408.
[102] Ibid., p. 570.
[103] Ibid., pp. 570 and 571.
[104] Monica Greco, 'Biopolitics, Psychosomatics, Participating Bodies', *Medical Humanities*, 45.2 (2019), 103–6.
[105] Jon Stone, 'What Should We Say to Patients with Symptoms Unexplained by Disease? The "Number Needed to Offend"', *BMJ*, 325.7378 (2002), 1449–50.
[106] Suzanne O'Sullivan, *It's All in Your Head: True Stories of Imaginary Illness* (London: Chatto & Windus, 2015), p. 81.

have been even more simple than hysterical autosuggestion: on the train home to Paris, Marie discovers a nail jutting out from her wheelchair that would have been pressing into her lower limb and causing her significant pain.[107] Despite this observation, the novel overwhelmingly affirms not only the connection between mind and body, but also the mysteriousness of that connection. If the nature of suffering may be mysteriously psychosomatic, the novel asks, then medicine must embrace alternative cures to find the best method of alleviating human suffering:

> Quel était donc cet impérieux besoin d'au-delà qui torturait l'humanité souffrante? D'où venait-il? [...] Toujours la soif inextinguible du bonheur l'avait brûlé, toujours elle le brûlerait. Si les pères de la Grotte faisaient de si glorieuses affaires, c'était qu'ils vendaient du divin. Cette soif du divin, que rien n'a pu étancher au travers des siècles, semblait renaître avec une violence nouvelle, au bout de notre siècle de science.[108]

> So what was this pressing need for the afterlife that tortured a suffering humanity? Where did it come from? [...] The unquenchable thirst for happiness had always burned him, and always would. If the priests of the Grotto did such brisk trade, it was because they sold the Divine. This thirst for the Divine, which nothing has been able to quench throughout the centuries, seemed to be reborn with a new violence at the end of our century of science.

In this passage, Pierre suggests that religion's popularity can be explained by how it answers fundamental questions relating to being and suffering. Medicine, he reasons, should compete with religion by similarly acknowledging the inexplicable and the unknown: 'Aujourd'hui l'expérience était faite, rien que la science ne semblait pouvoir suffire, et on allait être forcé de laisser une porte ouverte sur le mystère' ['Today the experiment was completed, nothing science could do seemed to be enough, and we had to leave the door open to mystery'].[109] This idea means that Pierre cannot take away Marie's faith since it helps alleviate her pain, although it also fails to inspire him to convert back to Catholicism. Pierre abandons the empirical truth of Beauclair's diagnosis and prediction in favour of the supernatural explanation to which Marie and the doctors subscribe. Although he cannot wholeheartedly subscribe to the doctors' religious-inspired medical opinion, Pierre decides to focus on the extent to which certification alleviates Marie's suffering.

Lourdes is productively understood in the context of *Le Docteur Pacal*, even though they belong to different novelistic cycles and, seemingly, to different

[107] Zola, *Lourdes*, p. 536.
[108] Ibid., p. 574.
[109] Ibid., p. 574.

phases of Zola's career. In *Le Docteur Pascal* we saw how the eponymous character attempts to forge a new, idealized form of medicine, and medical authority, through the *théorie dernière* that places the doctor at the heart of the medical relationship. Pascal dreams of a 'médecine nouvelle' ['new medicine'] in which the doctor possesses an 'autorité toute-puissante' ['all-powerful authority'] that allows him to heal his patients through their belief in his power rather than through the scientific exactitude of his methods.[110] In *Lourdes*, it is the doctor–patient relationship that is innovated: the novel imagines a new form of medicine that, through the embrace of the unknowns of medicine, the patient enjoys some form of healing. In this way, *Lourdes* anticipates psychosomatic medicine's mission to prioritize the embodied experience of illness over the pathological presence of disease, as well as recent calls to frame *medicine*, but not disorders, as psychosomatic in order to reaffirm the term's important contribution to the mind-body relationship whilst eschewing the potential impact of a derogatory term on patients.[111]

Reframing Marie's illness as one that resonates with current frameworks of psychosomatic medicine has consequences for how we interpret her marginalized position within the text. Lawrence Kirmayer and Ana Gómez-Carrillo outline how efforts to account for unexplained physical symptoms raise questions regarding the ascription of agency to the patient.[112] Residual forms of the mind/body dualism engender an ontology that ascribes agency to things that move on their own (such as breath or soul) as well as to the abstract concepts to which they give rise (such as the self). This framework allows for patients to perceive some intentions as full of agency and others as less so: for example, a patient may explain that they do not want to cry, although their body does.[113] In *Lourdes*, then, if Marie's body departs from her own will through its paralysis, itself informed and fuelled by the Marian cult as we saw previously, the character undergoes a reduction in agency. This limited personal agency is only amplified by the novel given the latter's focus on male characters' perceptions of Marie's illness, rather than her own embodied experience. However, the tension between mind and body in unexplained illnesses does not inevitably necessitate a reduction in agency. As pointed out already, the experience of mental and physical illness can be understood as offering a new form of power to otherwise disempowered patients and, as Thompson observes, this mechanism can be perceived in how Marie's body repels the doctor's medical gaze through the novel's sense of modesty. In short, the conceptual framework of

[110] Zola, *Le Docteur Pascal*, p. 376.

[111] Bryan Lask, '"Psychosomatic Medicine" Not "Psychosomatic Disorders"', *Journal of Psychosomatic Research*, 40.5 (1996), 457–60.

[112] Laurence J. Kirmayer and Ana Gómez-Carrillo, 'Agency, Embodiment and Enactment in Psychosomatic Theory and Practice', *Medical Humanities*, 45.2 (2019), 169–82.

[113] Ibid., p. 171.

psychosomatic medicine can inadvertently empower patients when the doctor–patient relationship is primed to embrace the mysterious aspects of illness and suffering.

Lourdes goes beyond this redemptive reading of the doctor–patient relationship by challenging the premises on which it is founded. Throughout the present study, we have seen that the doctor–patient relationship revolves around an asymmetric and binary interpersonal relationship (although these values are repeatedly questioned). Yet *Lourdes* radically re-conceives the doctor–patient relationship itself, anticipating recent calls made by critical medical humanities scholars to expand our narrow definition of medicine's primal scene to include other medical practitioners, as well as the friends and family of the patient.[114] Although retaining the binary characteristic seen throughout this volume, the new medical relationship conceptualized in *Lourdes* is mutual, reciprocal, and, most importantly, animated by characters who operate outside of the conventional roles of doctor and patient (as we briefly saw in Wolmar's doctor-esque role in *La Nouvelle Héloïse*). Before concluding, then, let us return to the initial premise of *Lourdes*: a priest who has lost his faith travels to the famous pilgrimage town. Pierre's lost faith finds it counterpart in Doctor Chassaigne, one of the doctors of the *bureau des constatations*, a medical man who renounces his belief in science and chooses to use his medical background to verify miracles. The relationship between these characters reappears throughout the novel and at once appears as a form of ironic satire, but also as an example of an alternative form of the hierarchical and asymmetric doctor–patient relationship that valorizes mutual understanding and reciprocal healing. Chassaigne is first introduced via the narrative frame that introduces the backstory of the family's trip to Lourdes. During the onset of Marie's illness, Pierre began to question his faith for the first time and found solace only in the doctor, one of his father's friends. Chassaigne is described as 'un médecin de réelle valeur, qui se renfermait modestement dans son rôle de praticien, ayant l'unique ambition de guérir' ['a doctor of true value, who modestly confined himself to his role of practitioner, with the sole ambition of curing [patients]'].[115] However, on the second day of the pilgrimage Pierre unexpectedly meets Chassaigne and discovers that his situation has greatly changed. The doctor recounts that his wife's and daughter's deaths, neither of which he could explain, undermined his desire to live in addition to his belief in the potential efficacy of medical science. Bereft of his family, Chassaigne affirms that he decided to give himself to God: 'Je me suis donné à Dieu, puisque Dieu seul peut me les rendre' ['I gave myself to God, since only God can give them back to me'].[116] Later in the novel, Chassaigne defends

[114] See for example Thomas R. Cole, Nathan S. Carlin, and Ronald A. Carson *Medical Humanities: An Introduction* (Cambridge: Cambridge University Press, 2017), pp. 26–40.
[115] Zola, *Lourdes*, p. 59.
[116] Ibid., p. 185.

the Grotto waters' healing potential given the current deficiencies in medical science.[117] This argument leads Pierre to understand Lourdes as an 'extraordinaire spectacle' ['extraordinary spectacle'].[118]

Despite the differences in opinion that the beginning of the novel emphasizes, Pierre and Chassaigne meet on a few occasions towards the end of *Lourdes* in a more conciliatory atmosphere. Chassaigne educates Pierre on Bernadette's own story, and these accounts compose the final chapter of the five sections that the novel is divided into. On the fourth day, Chassaigne takes Pierre's to Bernadette's abandoned room, the impoverished state of which, in contrast to the Grotto, causes Pierre to understand her unacknowledged importance to the town: 'l'idée leur était revenue que, sans Bernadette, rien n'aurait existé des prodiges qui avaient fait de Lourdes une ville unique au monde' ['the idea came to them that, without Bernadette, none of the miracles would have existed that had made Lourdes unique in the world'].[119] After Chassaigne argues that individual suffering tends to be the foundation for religion, Pierre is filled with pity and understanding for Bernadette:

> Si le rêve d'une enfant souffrante avait suffi pour amener les peuples, pour faire pleuvoir les millions et pousser du sol une cité nouvelle, n'était-ce pas que ce rêve venait apaiser un peu la faim des pauvres hommes, l'insatiable besoin qu'ils ont d'être trompés et consolés? Elle avait rouvert l'inconnu, sans doute à un moment social et historique favorable; et les foules s'y étaient précipitées. Oh! se réfugier dans le mystère, quand la réalité est si dure, s'en remettre au miracle, puisque la nature cruelle semble une longue injustice! Mais on a beau organiser l'inconnu, le réduire en dogmes, en faire des religions révélées, il n'y a toujours au fond que cet appel de la souffrance, ce cri de la vie, exigeant la santé, la joie, le bonheur fraternel, jusqu'à l'accepter dans un autre monde, s'il ne peut être sur cette terre. À quoi bon croire aux dogmes? Ne suffit-il pas de pleurer et d'aimer?[120]

> If the dream of a suffering child had been enough to bring people, to make millions come to Lourdes in their droves and to grow a new city from the ground, was it not that this dream had come to appease, a little bit, the hunger of poor men, the insatiable need they have to be deceived and consoled? Lourdes had reopened the unknown, no doubt at a favourable social and historical moment; and the crowds had rushed towards it. Oh! To take refuge in mystery when reality is so harsh, to rely on miracles since cruel nature feels like an enduring injustice! But try as we might to organize the unknown, reduce it into dogmas, turn it into religions, there is always only, deep down, this call of suffering, this cry of life,

[117] Ibid., pp. 212–13.
[118] Ibid., p. 214.
[119] Ibid., p. 437.
[120] Ibid., pp. 441–2.

> demanding health, joy, fraternal happiness, to the point of accepting it in another world, if it cannot take place on this earth. What is the use of believing in dogmas? Isn't it enough to cry and to love?

In this passage, we see the beginnings of the conclusion that Pierre will draw at the end of the novel regarding the importance of the *mystère* to the practice of medicine. Bernadette is described as opening the door onto the 'inconnu' that allows suffering to be appeased and the reality of life to be ignored momentarily. However, Zola here rails against the dogma of religion which is characterized as suffocating the genuine healing capacity of the *inconnu* (which heals through emotional recognition and reciprocity) and exploiting it for its own ends. In this way, Zola extricates faith from organized religion and finds value in the former that is otherwise extinguished by the latter.

As such, *Lourdes* forges an idea of reciprocal healing that is embodied in the unorthodox doctor–patient relationship that exists between Chassaigne and Pierre, who come to a shared understanding about Bernadette's role in the founding of Lourdes and, through this, enter into a pact of reciprocal and reflexive aide. The participants in this unconventional healing relationship also gain greater understanding regarding their own current crises of faith and the importance of capturing the *inconnu* and *mystère* whilst they continue their own personal journeys. This discourse of healing can apply to non-medical characters and expands our understanding of the genre of 'illness narrative'. Rereading Zola's *Lourdes* thus challenges us to expand our own conception of the doctor–patient relationship beyond the confines of the consultation room or the hospital, and instead to redefine it as a form of healing that heals not only the patient, but also medicine itself.

Conclusion

Zola's *Lourdes* illustrates how the medical encounter can understand, access, and harness the invisible forces that act on the body, incarnated in the new sciences of hysteria and microbes. The novel criticizes the Church for its apparent creation of religious hysteria, that contributes to, firstly, a mania for the Marian cult that manifests itself as a rejection of sexual reproduction and, secondly, an obsession for the holiness of the Grotto's waters that culminates in the neglect of basic hygiene protocols. The novel envisions a form of medicine that responds to these religious discourses by embracing the mysterious aspects of illness and the relationship between mind and body. Notwithstanding Zola's criticism of the role of medical doctors at Lourdes, the novel, through its use of water metaphors, suggests what religion and science have in common. Both rely on the belief in what cannot be seen with the naked eye, foregrounding the importance of subjective belief in the mysterious and the unknown. *Lourdes*'s criticism of the Marian cult is squarely aimed at its promotion of virginity over reproduction, an aim that ran counter to Zola's own natalist beliefs. Moreover, Pierre searches for a humane religion which seeks to alleviate suffering rather than promote it as a path to moral salvation. *Lourdes* presents the doctor–patient encounter to navigate these diverse themes and moral questions. Beauclair provides an example of how doctors can increase their medical and professional authority by remaining open to the mysteriousness of psychosomatic illnesses. Pierre, however, does not enjoy this luxury of professional detachment. Eventually he comes to understand that the relief of Marie's suffering, by whatever means and with whatever consequences, is more important than his search for truth.

By imagining contrasting but equally limited medical encounters, the novel contributes to a new conceptualization of the doctor–patient relationship. This medical relationship is focused primarily on healing and can either take a mutual form (such as that between Pierre and Chassaigne) or be asymmetric (such as between Beauclair and Marie, or even between Pierre and Marie). Furthermore, *Lourdes* questions the extent to which the conventional doctor–patient relationship is reliant on the presence of an afflicted patient and their attending doctor. By representing a doctor–patient relationship that allows for an embrace of the mysteriousness of the invisible forces that act within and without the body, *Lourdes* resonates with the concept of medicine formulated towards the end of *Le Docteur Pascal*, as we saw in Chapter One. Pascal's magical serum may, on the one hand, articulate Pascal's desire to end suffering through the advance of science; but, on the other hand, the serum's partial successes suggest that science can only go so far in providing the comfort required to alleviate suffering. *Lourdes* also challenges the pattern that we have seen elsewhere in the present study: whereas, in novels such as *Lamiel* and *Lélia*, the medical encounter is a site of resistance to the doctor–patient relationship; in *Lourdes* it is in fact the encounter that is seen as flawed. Indeed, the doctor–patient relationship then returns (in its new configuration) as an antidote to the limitations of the doctor–patient encounter. At the end of the century, then, *Lourdes* re-imagines the doctor–patient relationship in order to herald its return.

Conclusion

Doctors and Patients: Into the Twenty-First Century

How has the doctor–patient relationship changed since the nineteenth century? An answer to this question surely lies, at least in part, within the context of the history of medicine itself. For example, medical historians are now beginning to understand the full extent to which the influenza pandemic of 1918–20 altered the course of modern medicine.[1] Moreover, medicine's place in literary consciousness, has been brought to light only recently. As Elizabeth Outka argues in her study of the influence of the influenza pandemic on the development of English modernism, the doctor–patient relationship receded in importance to literary representations of medicine, which tended to focus on the experience of influenza itself.[2] In the twenty-first century, the coronavirus (COVID-19) pandemic forced a large-scale reckoning with how patients relate to their caregivers, how citizens relate to their politicians, as well as how global interconnectedness necessitates a broad view of public health and social relations. One of the most widely circulated 'good news' images during the coronavirus pandemic is that of healthcare workers in full PPE (personal protection equipment), attaching photos of themselves in their usual workwear attire to their suits to reassure their patients of their own humaneness.[3] In the spring of 2020, British healthcare workers were applauded weekly for what was styled by the Conservative government as their 'heroism'; but, ten weeks later, Annemarie Plas, the originator of 'Clap for our Carers', asked for the ritual to end due to its increasing politicization.[4] Since 2020, the changing status and importance of the doctor–patient relationship demonstrate the mercurial nature of modern medicine. What broader the present conclusions can be drawn from study of the representation of the doctor–patient relationship in the nineteenth-century French novel?

[1] Frank M. Snowden, *Epidemics and Society: From the Black Death to the Present* (New Haven, CT: Yale University Press, 2019), pp. 408–24.

[2] Elizabeth Outka, *Viral Modernism: The Influenza Pandemic and Interwar Literature* (New York: Columbia University Press, 2020).

[3] American Hospital Association, 'Health Care Workers in PPE Wear Photos of Themselves Smiling to Comfort Patients', https://www.aha.org/other-resources/2020-04-20-health-care-workers-ppe-wear-photos-themselves-smiling-comfort-patients.

[4] PA Media, 'Let's Stop Clapping for the NHS, Says Woman Who Started the Ritual', *The Guardian*, 22 May 2020 https://www.theguardian.com/world/2020/may/22/lets-stop-clapping-for-the-nhs-says-woman-who-started-the-ritual.

The Doctor–Patient Relationship and the Nineteenth-Century French Novel. Sarah Jones, Oxford University Press.
 DOI: 10.1093/oso/9780198893790.003.0006

As I have argued throughout the present study, the beginning of the nineteenth century was crucial in the development of modern medicine. Foucault outlines how Xavier Bichat's rediscovery of pathological anatomy created and ingrained the *regard médical*.[5] Foucault's argument has influenced medical historians such as Brockliss and Jones who have generally observed that nineteenth-century medicine was characterized by a distinct turn away from patient-centric medicine of the early modern period.[6] However, the *idea* of the doctor–patient relationship, and the imagined *experience* of the doctor–patient relationship, persisted in literature as an important trope through which authors represented medicine, regardless of whether they wished to worship at the altar of medical science or to criticize modern medicine and its practitioners.

In the context of nineteenth-century French literature, the doctor–patient relationship is a form of practice that hinges on an ongoing negotiation between doctor and patient that is both fluid and dynamic. Chapters One and Four outlined how the medical relationship can also be understood as an imagined ideal. These narratives focus on the character of the doctor: both Balzac's *Le Médecin de campagne* and Zola's *Le Docteur Pascal* venerate their eponymous medical characters for their benevolent approach to the doctor–patient relationship and their dedication to the local community but, at the same time, reveal the characters' personal and professional failures. In this respect, Chassaigne from Zola's *Lourdes* could also be included among doctor characters such as Pascal and Benassis given his attachment to his immediate community (which is an ever-changing stream of pilgrims rather than a stable rural community) as well as his attachment to the region of his birth to which he returns. The idealization of the doctor–patient relationship functions through the valorization of the doctor at the expense of the patient. Overall, in the novels in which the doctor–patient relationship is the dominant form of medical practice presented to the reader, the patient takes on a more passive characterization and role within the plot. We may think of the marginalized and dehumanized villagers of *Le Médecin de campagne*, the victims of Pascal's failed medical experiments, and the silenced voice of Marie in *Lourdes*. It cannot be overlooked that these relationships routinely consist of a male doctor and a patient from a marginalized group.

By contrast, the doctor–patient encounter represents an alternative experience of medicine. By their nature, novels such as *Le Médecin de campagne* and *Le Docteur Pascal* all contain medical encounters, but Chapters Two and Three of this study in particular highlight how this encounter can be a site of patient subversion and rebellion. In Stendhal's *Lamiel* and Sand's *Lélia*, the narrative focus shifts to the patient, even though the narrator may maintain an ambiguous stance

[5] Michel Foucault, *Naissance de la clinique* (Paris: Presses universitaires de France, 2017), p. 178.

[6] Laurence Brockliss and Colin Jones, *The Medical World of Early Modern France* (Oxford: Clarendon Press, 1997), pp. 819–24.

on doctor, as in the case of Sansfin in *Lamiel*, or outright satirize him, as in the case of Kreyssneifetter in *Lélia*. These subversive encounters focus on the female character's body, experience, and voice. In *Lélia* the eponymous female patient is presented as unreadable, and Marie's sense of *pudeur* and her thinness may create a similar effect in *Lourdes*. In both *Lélia* and *Lamiel*, the female patient is presented as rebellious and, through either manipulating iconography associated with femininity or through a pastiche of Balzacian literature, she is characterized as coming into self-knowledge and self-possession at the very moment of the medical encounter, thereby inverting the ordinarily hierarchical, asymmetric, and binary doctor–patient relationship. The fact that these texts have rarely been read as illness narratives also expands our present understanding of the genre and forges a new role for literary studies within it. The voices of these female patient characters are either central to their respective novels, particularly in the case of our eponymous heroines, or are marginalized as in the case of *Lourdes*.

However, the terms doctor–patient relationship and encounter are neither antithetical nor mutually exclusive. The doctor–patient relationship and encounter are connected temporally and thus enjoy a symbiotic and fluid relationship with one another. As I have emphasized throughout, some novels may favour either the doctor–patient relationship or encounter, but they can represent both the medical relationship and encounter, further pointing towards the slippage inherent in these two terms. Chapter One focused on the idealized form of the doctor–patient relationship which was made up of a number of highly charged medical encounters. Stendhal's *Lamiel* depicts the eponymous heroine's ongoing relationship with her doctor, but in Chapter Two I demonstrated that it uses a singular doctor–patient encounter to upend the dynamics of that relationship. Chapter Three extended this function of the doctor–patient encounter: Lélia seems to have no prior relationship with Kreyssneifetter before her bedside consultation with him, and he does not appear later in the novel. *Lourdes* is perhaps the most ambiguous text when seen from this perspective: Chapter Four demonstrated that Marie has a series of one-off encounters with her eminent Parisian doctors, including Beauclair, as well as the doctors of the *bureau de constatations*. Yet Pierre's ongoing relationships with Beauclair and Chassaigne suggest that the novel offers a new form of healing doctor–patient relationship that replaces what is represented as the dysfunctional medical encounter. From these characterizations, the doctor–patient relationship in the nineteenth century tends to be a form of power or authority associated with masculine characters and their plots, whereas the doctor–patient encounter shines light on female characters and their resistance to medical forms of knowledge. Future studies could productively explore how female, non-binary, or gender-fluid medical characters affect the representation of the doctor–patient relationships.

Literary representations of the doctor–patient relationship bring abstract, immaterial, and self-reflexive concerns regarding power and knowledge into dialogue with the concrete, material, and unavoidable aspects of illness and death. The waxing and waning of the doctor–patient relationship reflects how these concerns, divided between the material and the immaterial, are negotiated between doctor and patient in the novel. This process of negotiation allows an incorporation of a range of medical discourse into literary works, as well as responses to them. The doctor–patient encounter is one such response since it is almost always a particularly important dramatic moment in which these questions are explored and negotiated. Exploring the cleavage between the ideal medical relationship and encounter is a central occupation of the novel in this period. The fluid nature of the doctor–patient relationship also points to the possibility of new conceptions of literary depictions of medical practice in the nineteenth-century novel: how do other medical practitioners and caregivers interact with patients, and what does this change about the experience of being ill?

The doctor–patient relationship and encounter are particularly interesting paradigms since they throw light on the perennial question of whether medicine is best understood as a science or art.[7] On the one hand, and from the perspective that resonates most strongly with conceptions of medicine after the development of microbiology, medicine is governed by scientific principles and studies. In this sense, the inclusion of medicine in narrative allows authors to situate medicine within its scientific intellectual context. It is for this reason that the present book has adopted a historicist approach that has allowed for the comparing of literary narratives to contemporary medical treatises and documents. On the other hand, medicine could also be seen as reflecting the practices commonly found within literary studies, such as the analogy commonplace in the medical humanities between literary narrative and illness narrative, and thus the idea that the doctor should learn to 'read' the patient. However, this study has argued that the nineteenth-century French novel responds to this dichotomous way of understanding medicine by suggesting a third option. The doctor–patient relationship and encounter draw attention to how novels represent or rather imagine a form of medicine that is being practiced and experienced. Yet the nature of that practice differs depending on whether the novel favours either the idealized doctor–patient relationship or the subversive medial encounter. For idealized doctor characters, medicine is a duty that is performed, an examination that is completed, a treatment that is administered, a cure that is sought; for their patients, medicine is something that is enthusiastically received. But for novels that favour depictions of the doctor–patient encounter, the doctor is characterized as attempting to control the patient, or even to harm them; the patient, in turn, may try to resist them by questioning the bases on which their authority is founded.

As Whitehead observes, the role of literary studies and literature within the medical humanities is often restricted to an 'additive' function that enriches or

[7] Gavin Francis, 'Medicine: Art or Science?', *The Lancet*, 395.10217 (2020), 24–5.

reinforces the current practice of medicine.[8] This study has attempted to go beyond this position by challenging critical assumptions about, and approaches to, the doctor–patient relationship, building on Elsner's observation that literary texts can resist power structures and abstract concepts on a textual level.[9] Further, it has foregrounded that literary forms themselves are what undermines these notions: it is thanks to the ambiguity, ambivalence, and slipperiness of literary language that the complex interplay between medical relationship and encounter is revealed. The present study has thus strived to be a form of critique of, and resistance to, normative ways of approaching both medicine and the medical humanities, helping bring the medical humanities closer towards a more global, and thus linguistically diverse, approach to medicine and illness.

The critical medical humanities have recently become more interested in fragmented or avant-garde forms of literature, arguing that such abstractions challenge the assumptions that underpin the practice of modern medicine. Yet nineteenth-century texts also participate in this dismantling of the structures and hierarchies of medicine (indeed, as much as they reinforce and perpetuate them). Where some scholars encourage the medical humanities to move beyond realist texts and to embrace non-narrative forms, I instead argue these texts challenge practices surrounding medicine, and that they do so through both the complex nature of realist literary modes and realism's interconnection with idealism. Literary features such as metaphor, narrative perspective, and plot are both central to this argument. To take only the example of medical plots, Brooks argues that nineteenth-century novels are characterized by their interest and investment in plot, connected to both desire and time. Moving beyond this analogy between realism and the *regard médical*, the novel's emphasis on practice explains the position that medicine (in the form of medical scenes and characters, as well as illness and death) enjoys. Moreover, the difference between the doctor–patient relationship and encounter is best understood as a temporal one, and temporality itself is responsible for 'the motor forces that drive the text forward, [...] the desires that connect narrative ends and beginnings, and make of the textual middle a highly charged field of force'.[10] The introduction of medicine into a novel allows plot to function: the threat of illness or death, or the potential harmful actions of a nefarious doctor, accelerates the novel's inevitable movement towards its own end and thence to death. In extreme cases, such as in *Lamiel*, the doctor may even explicitly delight in the patient's death:

[8] Anne Whitehead, 'The Medical Humanities: A Literary Perspective', in *Medicine, Health and the Arts: Approaches to the Medical Humanities*, ed. by Victoria Bates, Alan Bleakley, and Sam Goodman (London: Routledge, 2013), p. 7.

[9] Anna Magdalena Elsner, 'Beyond Medical Paternalism: Undoing the Doctor-Patient Relationship in Simone de Beauvoir's A Very Easy Death', *Literature and Medicine*, 37.2 (2019), p. 422.

[10] Peter Brooks, *Reading for the Plot: Design and Intention in Narrative* (Cambridge, MA; London: Harvard University Press, 1992), pp. xiii–xiv.

> On vint le chercher [Sansfin] pour un beau jeune homme de cnq pieds six pouces et qui ventait, à peine âgè de vingt-cinq ans, d'avoir une belle et bonne attaque d'apoplexie. Le docteur passa la nuit auprès de lui, et, tout en lui appliquant le traitement convenable, il eut le plaisir de voir cet être si beau mourir avec la pointe du jour.[11]

> [Sansfin] was fetched for a handsome young man of five feet six inches, who had just suffered a massive stroke at the age of twenty five. The doctor spent the night with him and, while administering the appropriate treatment, he had the pleasure of seeing this beautiful creature die with the dawn.

In this passage, Sansfin sadistically enjoys his patient's death, and the narration focalized through his eyes draws attention to the 'belle et bonne' condition from which the patient suffers. By emphasizing what medicine can do for texts from the perspective of narrative, and by recreating the medical, cultural, and sociopolitical contexts of the nineteenth-century novel, French fiction's interest in the doctor–patient encounter lies in its ability to narrativize themes and discourses in contemporary medicine by embedding it into plot, characterization, and thematic constructs. As Porter observes, it is 'people and cultures [that] have always given meaning to disease', and literature's emphasis on plot and narrative doubtlessly increases its contribution to the breadth of meaning that both illness and medicine enjoy.[12] The texts discussed in this monograph are potentially useful to scholars in the medical humanities, as well as students and practitioners of medicine, since they draw attention to the multiplicity and plurality of medical practice and the ways that narrative intervenes within these negotiations. I hope that this volume has inspired readers to think beyond the concept of the doctor–patient relationship as well as to interrogate its form, function, and significance. By uncovering the interpersonal dynamic inherent in medicine, the reader can perhaps perceive afresh the personal, experiential, and embodied interactions and metaphors embedded within systems of discursive knowledge and power beyond the medical context.

[11] Stendhal, *ORC*, III, p. 989.

[12] Roy Porter and G. S. Rousseau, *Gout: The Patrician Malady* (New Haven, CT; London: Yale University Press, 1998), p. 285.

Bibliography

Ackerknecht, Erwin H., *Medicine at the Paris Hospital, 1794–1848* (Baltimore, MD: Johns Hopkins Press, 1967)

American Hospital Association, 'Health Care Workers in PPE Wear Photos of Themselves Smiling to Comfort Patients', *American Hospital Association*, <https://www.aha.org/other-resources/2020-04-20-health-care-workers-ppe-wear-photos-themselves-smiling-comfort-patients>

Andréoli, Max, 'Morale de la politique et politique de la morale dans *La Comédie humaine*', *L'Année balzacienne*, 4.1 (2003), 125–60 <https://doi.org/10.3917/balz.004.0125>

Ansel, Yves, *Stendhal littéral: 'Lamiel'* (Grenoble: ELLUG, 2009)

Armstrong, David, 'Bodies of Knowledge / Bodies of Power', in *Reassessing Foucault: Power, Medicine, and the Body*, ed. by Colin Jones and Roy Porter (London; New York: Routledge, 1994), pp. 17–27

Arrambide, J. B., *Explication des symptômes du cholera-morbus, des apparences cadavériques, et de ses méthodes curatives, par des données physiologiques* (Paris: Éverat, 1832)

Athanassoglou-Kallmyer, Nina, 'Blemished Physiologies: Delacroix, Paganini, and the Cholera Epidemic of 1832', *The Art Bulletin*, 83.4 (2001), 686–710.

Bachelard, Gaston, *L'Eau et les rêves: essai sur l'imagination de la matière* (Paris: J. Corti, 1963)

Bachelard, Gaston, *La Formation de l'esprit scientifique: contribution à une psychanalyse de la connaissance objective* (Paris: Librairie J. Vrin, 2000)

Baguley, David, 'Du récit polémique au discours utopique: l'Évangile républicain de Zola', *Cahiers naturalistes*, 54 (1980), 106–21

Baguley, David, *Naturalist Fiction: The Entropic Vision* (Cambridge: Cambridge University Press, 1990)

Bailey, Peter, *The New Doctor, Patient, Illness Model: Restoring the Authority of the GP Consultation* (London: Radcliffe Publishing, 2014)

Balint, Michael, *The Doctor, His Patient, and the Illness*, with an Introduction by John A. Balint (Edinburgh: Churchill Livingstone, 2000)

Balzac, Honoré de, *Correspondance*, ed. by Roger Pierrot and Hervé Yon, 3 vols (Paris: Gallimard, 2006–11)

Balzac, Honoré de, *Le Cousin Pons*, ed. by Jacques Thuillier and André Lorant (Paris: Gallimard, 2007)

Balzac, Honoré de, *La Cousine Bette*, ed. by Pierre Barbéris (Paris: Gallimard, 1973)

Balzac, Honoré de, *Le Médecin de campagne*, ed. by Jean A. Ducourneau (Paris: Livre de Poche, 1966)

Balzac, Honoré de, *La Muse du département; Un prince de la bohème*, ed. by Patrick Berthier (Paris: Gallimard, 2007)

Balzac, Honoré de, *La Peau de chagrin*, ed. by Nadine Satiat (Paris: Flammarion, 1996)

Balzac, Honoré de, *Le Père Goriot*, ed. by Félicien Marceau (Paris: Gallimard, 1971)

Balzac, Honoré de, *Les Secrets de la princesse de Cadignan et autres études de femme*, ed. by Samuel S. de Sacy and Jean Roudaut (Paris: Gallimard, 1980)

Balzac, Honoré de, *Une double famille, suivi du Contrat de mariage et de L'Interdiction*, ed. by Samuel S. de Sacy (Paris: Gallimard, 1973)

Barker, Emma, 'Reading the Greuze Girl: The Daughter's Seduction', *Representations*, 117.1 (2012), 86–119 <https://doi.org/10.1525/rep.2012.117.1.86>

Barnes, David S., *The Making of a Social Disease: Tuberculosis in Nineteenth-Century France* (Berkeley, CA; London: University of California Press, 1995)

Baron, Anne-Marie, 'Balzac et le *Contrat social* de Rousseau', *L'Année balzacienne*, 11.1 (2010), 249–65 <https://doi.org/10.3917/balz.011.0249>

Barthes, Roland, 'L'Effet de réel', *Communications*, 11.1 (1968), 84–9 <https://doi.org/10.3406/comm.1968.1158>

Beauvoir, Simone de, *Le Deuxième Sexe: les faits et les mythes*, 2 vols (Paris: Gallimard, 2012)

Beizer, Janet L., *Ventriloquized Bodies: Narratives of Hysteria in Nineteenth-Century France* (Ithaca, NY: Cornell University Press, 1994)

Bell, Rudolph M., *Holy Anorexia* (Chicago, IL; London: University of Chicago Press, 1985)

Bennati and Miquel, 'Notice physiologique sur Paganini', *Revue de Paris*, 26 (1831), 52–60

Berger, John, *A Fortunate Man: The Story of a Country Doctor* (Edinburgh: Canongate, 2016)

Berthier, Philippe, *Lamiel, ou, La Boîte de Pandore* (Paris: Presses universitaires de France, 1994)

Bertrand, Alexandre, 'Rapport secret sur le magnétisme, par Bailly et ses collègues', in *Du magnétisme animal en France* (Paris: J. Baillère, 1826), pp. 511–16

Billington, Josie, *Is Literature Healthy?* (Oxford: Oxford University Press, 2016)

Bleakley, Alan, *Educating Doctors' Senses through the Medical Humanities: 'How Do I Look?'* (Abingdon; New York: Routledge, 2020)

Boutry, Philippe, 'Marie, la grande consolatrice de la France au XIXème siècle', *L'Histoire*, 50 (1982), 31–9

British Medical Association, 'Requirement for All Patients to Have a Named GP', *BMA*, 7 September 2020, <https://www.bma.org.uk/advice-and-support/gp-practices/managing-your-practice-list/requirement-for-all-patients-to-have-a-named-gp>

Brockliss, Laurence and Colin Jones, *The Medical World of Early Modern France* (Oxford: Clarendon Press, 1997)

Brombert, Victor, *Stendhal: Fiction and the Themes of Freedom* (Chicago, IL: University of Chicago Press, 1976)

Brookner, Anita, *Greuze: The Rise and Fall of an Eighteenth-Century Phenomenon* (London: Elek, 1972)

Brooks, Peter, *Body Work: Objects of Desire in Modern Narrative* (Cambridge, MA: Harvard University Press, 1993)

Brooks, Peter, 'The Novel and the Guillotine; or, Fathers and Sons in *Le Rouge et le Noir*', *PMLA*, 97.3 (1982), 348–62 <https://doi.org/10.2307/462227>

Brooks, Peter, *Reading for the Plot: Design and Intention in Narrative* (Cambridge, MA; London: Harvard University Press, 1992)

Brumberg, Joan Jacobs, *Fasting Girls: The History of Anorexia Nervosa* (New York: Vintage, 2000)

Cabanès, Jean-Louis, *Le Corps et la maladie dans les récits réalistes (1856–1893)*, 2 vols (Paris: Klincksieck, 1991)

Cabanis, Pierre-Jean-Georges, *Du Degré de certitude de la médecine* (Paris: Crapat & Ravier, 1803)

Charcot, Jean-Martin, *La Foi qui guérit* (Paris: Félix Alcan, 1897)

Charcot, Jean-Martin, *Leçons sur les maladies du système nerveux*, 3 vols (Paris: Lecrosnieret Babé, 1890)

Charon, Rita, *Narrative Medicine: Honoring the Stories of Illness* (New York; Oxford: Oxford University Press, 2006)

Chéron, Jules, *Introduction à l'étude des lois générales de l'hypodermie, physiologie et thérapeutique* (Paris: Société d'éditions scientifiques, 1893)

Chipidza, Fallon E., Rachel S. Wallwork, and Theodore A. Stern, 'Impact of the Doctor–Patient Relationship', *The Primary Care Companion for CNS Disorders*, 17.5 (2015) <https://doi.org/10.4088/PCC.15f01840>

Chiron, Yves, *Enquête sur les miracles de Lourdes* (Paris: Perrin, 2008)

Chua, Kevin, 'Dead Birds, or the Miseducation of the Greuze Girl', in *Performing the 'Everyday': The Culture of Genre in the Eighteenth Century*, ed. by Alden Cavanaugh (Newark, DE: University of Delaware Press, 2007), pp. 75–91

Cole, Thomas R., Nathan S. Carlin, and Ronald A. Carson, *Medical Humanities: An Introduction* (Cambridge: Cambridge University Press, 2017)

Comfort, Kathleen Ann, 'Divine Images of Hysteria in Emile Zola's *Lourdes*', *Nineteenth-Century French Studies*, 30.3/4 (2002), 329–45

Corrado Pope, Barbara, 'Immaculate and Powerful: The Marian Revival in the Nineteenth Century', in *Immaculate and Powerful: The Female in Sacred and Social Reality*, ed. by Clarissa W. Atkinson, Constance H. Buchanan, and Margaret R. Miles (Wellingborough: Crucible, 1987), pp. 185–92

Counter, Andrew J., '*L'Interdiction*, or, Balzac on the Margins of Law and Realism', *Law and Humanities*, 11.1 (2017), 24–43 <https://doi.org/10.1080/17521483.2017.1320035>

Counter, Andrew J., 'Zola's *fin-de-siècle* Reproductive Politics', *French Studies*, 68.2 (2014), 193–208 <https://doi.org/10.1093/fs/knt302>

Crabtree, Adam, *From Mesmer to Freud: Magnetic Sleep and the Roots of Psychological Healing* (New Haven, CT; London: Yale University Press, 1993)

Crouzet, Michel, 'Le Dépucelage de Lamiel', in *Amicitia scriptor: littérature, histoire des idées, philosophie. Mélanges offerts à Robert Mauzi*, ed. by Annie Becq, Charles Porset, and Alain Mothu (Paris: Champion, 1998), pp. 293–313

Cryle, Peter, 'Foretelling Pathology: The Poetics of Prognosis', *French Cultural Studies*, 17.1 (2006), 107–22 <https://doi.org/10.1177/0957155806060799>

Cryle, Peter, 'Le Marbre féminin', *Revue des sciences humaines*, 271 (2003), 147–55

Cryle, Peter and Alison Moore, *Frigidity: An Intellectual History* (Basingstoke: Palgrave Macmillan, 2011)

Delaporte, François, *Disease and Civilization: The Cholera in Paris, 1832*, trans. by Arthur Goldhammer (Cambridge, MA; London: MIT Press, 1986)

Diaz, José-Luis, 'Balzac romancier de la "grande maladie sociale" (1838–1847)', *L'Année balzacienne*, 17.1 (2016), 221–40 <https://doi.org/10.3917/balz.017.0221>

Le Dictionnaire de l'Académie française (Paris: Brunet, 1762), s.v. 'puberté'

Le Dictionnaire de l'Académie française (Paris: J. J. Smits et Ce, 1798), s.v. 'science'

Le Dictionnaire de l'Académie française (Paris: Firmin Didot Frères, 1832), s.v. 'médecine'

Le Dictionnaire de l'Académie française (Paris: Didot, 1835), s.v. 'puberté'

Le Dictionnaire de l'Académie française (Paris: Hachette, 1935), s.v. 'science'

Diderot, Denis, *Salons* (Paris: Gallimard, 2008)

Didi-Huberman, Georges, *Invention de l'hystérie: Charcot et l'iconographie photographique de la Salpêtrière* (Paris: Macula, 1982)

Dijkstra, Bram, *Idols of Perversity: Fantasies of Feminine Evil in Fin-de-Siècle Culture* (New York: Oxford University Press, 1988)

Donaldson-Evans, Mary, *Medical Examinations: Dissecting the Doctor in French Narrative Prose, 1857–1894* (Lincoln, NE: University of Nebraska Press, 2000)

Douglas, Mary, *Purity and Danger: An Analysis of the Concepts of Pollution and Taboo* (London; New York: Routledge, 2005)

Downing, Lisa, *Desiring the Dead: Necrophilia and Nineteenth-Century French Literature* (Oxford: Legenda, 2003)

Duffin, Jacalyn, *To See with a Better Eye: A Life of R. T. H. Laennec* (Princeton, NJ; Chichester: Princeton University Press, 1998)

Duffy, Larry, *Flaubert, Zola, and the Incorporation of Disciplinary Knowledge* (Basingstoke; New York: Palgrave Macmillan, 2015)

Duffy, Larry, 'Medical Humanism or *Scientia Sexualis*? Building a Sexological Concept in *Fécondité*', *Nottingham French Studies*, 60.3 (2021) 317–33 <https://doi.org/10.3366/nfs.2021.0328>

Dunn, Michael, 'At the Moral Margins of the Doctor–Patient Relationship', *Journal of Medical Ethics*, 45.3 (2019), 149–50 <https://doi.org/10.1136/medethics-2019-105407>

Ellenberger, Henri F., *The Discovery of the Unconscious: The History and Evolution of Dynamic Psychiatry* (London: Fontana, 1994)

Elsner, Anna Magdalena, 'Beyond Medical Paternalism: Undoing the Doctor–Patient Relationship in Simone de Beauvoir's *A Very Easy Death*', *Literature and Medicine*, 37.2 (2019), 420–41 <https://doi.org/10.1353/lm.2019.0019>

Emanuel, Ezekiel J. and Linda L. Emanuel, 'Four Models of the Physician–Patient Relationship', *JAMA: The Journal of the American Medical Association*, 267.16 (1992), 2221 <https://doi.org/10.1001/jama.1992.03480160079038>

Evans, Richard J., *Death in Hamburg: Society and Politics in the Cholera Years, 1830–1910* (New York: Penguin Books, 2005)

Fabre, Antoine François Hippolyte, *Du choléra morbus de Paris; ou, guide des praticiens dans la connaissance et le traitement de cette maladie* (Paris: Germer Baillière, 1832)

Finn, Michael R., 'Doctors, Malady, and Creativity in Rachilde', *Nineteenth-Century French Studies*, 34.1–2 (2005), 121–33

Flaubert, Gustave, *Correspondance*, ed. by Jean Bruneau, 5 vols (Paris: Gallimard, 1973–2007)

Flaubert, Gustave, *Madame Bovary*, ed. by Thierry Laget (Paris: Gallimard, 2009)

Fort, Bernadette, 'The Greuze Girl: The Invention of a Pictorial Paradigm', *Studies in the History of Art*, 72 (2008), 128–51

Foucault, Michel, *Histoire de la sexualité*, 4 vols, (Paris: Gallimard, 1994)

Foucault, Michel, *Naissance de la clinique* (Paris: Presses universitaires de France, 2017)

Francis, Gavin, 'Medicine: Art or Science?', *The Lancet*, 395.10217 (2020), 24–5 <https://doi.org/10.1016/S0140-6736(19)33145-9>

Frank, Arthur W., *The Wounded Storyteller: Body, Illness, and Ethics* (Chicago, IL: University of Chicago Press, 2013)

Furlong, Monica, *Visions and Longings: An Anthology of Women Mystics* (London: Mowbray, 1996)

Furst, Lilian R., 'Realism and Hypertrophy: A Study of Three Medico-Historical "Cases"', *Nineteenth-Century French Studies*, 22.1/2 (1993), 29–47

Gadamer, Hans-Georg, *The Enigma of Health: The Art of Healing in a Scientific Age* (Stanford, CA: Stanford University Press, 1996)

Garnier, Lucy, 'La Femme comme construction dans la fiction stendhalienne' (DPhil thesis, University of Oxford, 2007)

Gawande, Atul, *Being Mortal: Illness, Medicine and What Matters in the End* (London: Profile Books, 2014)

Geisler-Szmulewicz, Anne, *Le Mythe de Pygmalion au XIXe siècle: pour une approche de la coalescence des mythes* (Paris: Honoré Champion, 1999)

Genette, Gérard, *Figures II* (Paris: Seuil, 1979)

Gerwin, Elisabeth, 'Le Mal du narcissisme chez Balzac', *L'Année balzacienne*, 17.1 (2016), 325–42 <https://doi.org/10.3917/balz.017.0325>

Goodman, Elise, '"Les Jeux innocents": French Rococo Birding and Fishing Scenes', *Simiolus: Netherlands Quarterly for the History of Art*, 23.4 (1995), 251–67 <https://doi.org/10.2307/3780798>

Goold, Susan Dorr and Mack Lipkin, 'The Doctor–Patient Relationship: Challenges, Opportunities, and Strategies', *Journal of General Internal Medicine*, 14.S1 (1999), S26–S33 <https://doi.org/10.1046/j.1525-1497.1999.00267.x>

Gosme, Michel, 'Le Nouveau statut de la science dans *Les Trois Villes*', *Cahiers naturalistes*, 74 (2000), 223–36

Goubert, Jean-Pierre, *La Conquête de l'eau: l'avènement de la santé à l'âge industriel* (Paris: R. Laffont, 1986)

Goulet, Andrea, *Optiques: The Science of the Eye and the Birth of Modern French Fiction* (Philadelphia, PA: University of Pennsylvania Press, 2006)

Greco, Monica, 'Biopolitics, Psychosomatics, Participating Bodies', *Medical Humanities*, 45.2 (2019), 103–6 <https://doi.org/10.1136/medhum-2019-011717>

Grosz, Elizabeth, *Volatile Bodies: Toward a Corporeal Feminism* (Bloomington, IN: Indiana University Press, 1994)

Harkness, Nigel, *Men of Their Words: The Poetics of Masculinity in George Sand's Fiction* (London: Legenda, 2007)

Harkness, Nigel, 'Resisting Realist Petrification in George Sand's *Lélia* and Balzac's *Sarrasine*', *French Studies*, 59.2 (2005), 159–72 <https://doi.org/10.1093/fs/kni136>

Harrow, Susan, *Zola, the Body Modern: Pressures and Prospects of Representation* (London: Legenda, 2010)

Hemmings, F. W. J, *Émile Zola* (Oxford: Clarendon Press, 1966)

Howells, R. J., *Rousseau, Julie ou la Nouvelle Héloïse* (London; Wolfeboro, NH: Grant & Cutler, 1986)

Hunt, Lynn, *The Family Romance of the French Revolution* (London: Routledge, 1992)

Hunter, Kathryn Montgomery, *Doctors' Stories: The Narrative Structure of Medical Knowledge* (Princeton, NJ: Princeton University Press, 1991)

Hurwitz, Brian and Victoria Bates, 'The Roots and Ramifications of Narrative in Modern Medicine', in *The Edinburgh Companion to the Critical Medical Humanities*, ed. by Anne Whitehead and Angela Woods (Edinburgh: University of Edinburgh Press, 2016), pp. 559–76

Huysmans, Joris-Karl, *Les Foules de Lourdes* (Paris: Stock, 1906)

Illich, Ivan, *Limits to Medicine. Medical Nemesis: The Expropriation of Health* (London: Calder & Boyars, 1975)

Israël, Lucien, *L'Hystérique, le sexe et le médecin* (Paris: Masson, 2001)

Jewson, N. D., 'The Disappearance of the Sick-Man from Medical Cosmology, 1770–1870', *International Journal of Epidemiology*, 38.3 (2009), 622–33 <https://doi.org/10.1093/ije/dyp180>

Jurecic, Ann, *Illness as Narrative* (Pittsburgh, PA: University of Pittsburgh Press, 2012)

Kirmayer, Laurence J., 'Broken Narratives: Clinical Encounters and the Poetics of Illness Experience', in *Narrative and the Cultural Construction of Illness and Healing*, ed. by Cheryl Mattingly and Linda C. Garro (Berkeley, CA: University of California Press, 2000), pp. 153–80

Kirmayer, Laurence J. and Ana Gómez-Carrillo, 'Agency, Embodiment and Enactment in Psychosomatic Theory and Practice', *Medical Humanities*, 45.2 (2019), 169–82 <https://doi.org/10.1136/medhum-2018-011618>

Kleinman, Arthur, *The Illness Narratives: Suffering, Healing and the Human Condition* (New York: Basic Books, 1988)

Knight, Diana, 'Conjugal Secrets in Balzac's *La Muse du département*', *Nineteenth-Century French Studies*, 40.3–4 (2012), 273–86 <https://doi.org/10.1353/ncf.2012.0000>

Konkin, Jill, Laura Grave, Ella Cockburn, and others, 'Exploration of Rural Physicians' Lived Experience of Practising Outside Their Usual Scope of Practice to Provide Access to Essential Medical Care (Clinical Courage): An International Phenomenological Study', *BMJ Open*, 10.8 (2020), e037705 <https://doi.org/10.1136/bmjopen-2020-037705>

Kristeva, Julia, *Pouvoirs de l'horreur: essai sur l'abjection* (Paris: Seuil, 1980)

Kristeva, Julia, *The Severed Head: Capital Visions*, trans. by Jody Gladding (New York: Columbia University Press, 2014)

Kristeva, Julia, Marie Rose Moro, John Ødemark, and Eivind Engebretsen, 'Cultural Crossings of Care: An Appeal to the Medical Humanities', *Medical Humanities*, 44.1 (2018), 55–8 <https://doi.org/10.1136/medhum-2017-011263>

Labourct, Mireille, 'De l'*Imitation de Jésus-Christ* à "l'évangile en action": images et paraboles dans *Le Médecin de campagne*', *L'Année balzacienne*, 4.1 (2003), 43–62 <https://doi.org/10.3917/balz.004.0043>

Laënnec, René-Théophile-Hyacinthe, *Traité de l'auscultation médiate, ou traité du diagnostic des maladies des poumons et du cœur*, 2 vols (Paris: J.-A. Brosson and J.-S. Chaudé, 1819)

Laënnec, René-Théophile-Hyacinthe, *Traité de l'auscultation médiate et des maladies des poumons et du cœur*, 2 vols (Paris: J.-S. Chaudé, 1826)

The Lancet, 'The Doctor–Patient Relationship: Capturing the Ideal', *The Lancet*, 381.9876, 27 April 2013, 1432 <https://doi.org/10.1016/S0140-6736(13)60911-3>

Lask, Bryan, '"Psychosomatic Medicine" Not "Psychosomatic Disorders"', *Journal of Psychosomatic Research*, 40.5 (1996), 457–60 <https://doi.org/10.1016/0022-3999(95)00578-1>

Latour, Bruno, *Les Microbes: guerre et paix; suivi de, Irréductions* (Paris: A. M. Métailié, 1984)

Lefevre, Anne-Marie, 'Bianchon, un astre du cosmos balzacien', *L'Année balzacienne*, 16 (1995), 311–50

Léonard, Jacques, *La Vie quotidienne du médecin de province au XIXe siècle* (Paris: France Loisirs, 1993)

Leroy, Sophie, 'Introduction', in *Medicine and Maladies: Representing Affliction in Nineteenth-Century France*, ed. by Sophie Leroy (Leiden: Brill, 2018), pp. 1–15 <https://doi.org/10.1163/9789004368019_002>

Le Yaouanc, Moïse, *Nosographie de l'humanité balzacienne* (Paris: Librairie Maloine, 1959)

Magendie, François, *Leçons sur le choléra-morbus* (Paris: Collège de France, 1832)

Manzini, Francesco, 'Doctors, Priests, Magistrates: Stendhal, Cabanis and the Power of Medical Practitioners', in *Institutions and Power in Nineteenth-Century French Literature and Culture*, ed. by David Evans and Kate Griffiths (Leiden: Brill, 2011), pp. 167–82 <https://doi.org/10.1163/9789401200806_012>

Marceau, Félicien, *Balzac et son monde* (Paris: Gallimard, 1986)

Marcus, Melissa, *The Representation of Mesmerism in Honoré de Balzac's La Comédie humaine* (New York: Peter Lang, 1995)

Mathias, Manon, *Vision in the Novels of George Sand* (Oxford: Oxford University Press, 2016)

Matlock, Jann, *Scenes of Seduction: Prostitution, Hysteria, and Reading Difference in Nineteenth-Century France* (New York: Columbia University Press, 1994)

Maupassant, Guy de, *Le Horla*, ed. by André Fermigier (Paris: Gallimard, 2009)

Mazaheri, John, *Essais sur la religiosité d'Honoré de Balzac* (Lewiston: Edwin Mellen Press, 2008)

McCaffrey, Enda and Áine Larkin, Introduction to *The Critical Medical Humanities*, ed. by Enda McCaffrey and Áine Larkin (special issue, *Essays in French Literature and Culture*, 58 (2021)), 3–14

McCaffrey, Enda and Steven Wilson, 'Introduction: Death and/as Relationality', in *French Thanatology*, ed. by Enda McCaffrey and Steven Wilson (special issue, *L'Esprit Créateur*, 61.1 (2021)), 1–12 <https://doi.org/10.1353/esp.2021.0000>

McEachern, Patricia A., '"La Vierge et La Bête": Marian Iconographies and Bestial Effigies in Nineteenth-Century French Narratives', *Nineteenth-Century French Studies*, 31.1/2 (2002), 111–22

Mesmer, Franz Anton, *Mémoire sur la découverte du magnétisme animal* (Genève: Didot, 1779)

Micale, Mark S., *Approaching Hysteria: Disease and Its Interpretations* (Princeton, NJ: Princeton University Press, 1994)

Micale, Mark S., *Hysterical Men: The Hidden History of Male Nervous Illness* (Cambridge, MA; London: Harvard University Press, 2008)

Micale, Mark S., *The Mind of Modernism: Medicine, Psychology, and the Cultural Arts in Europe and America, 1880–1940* (Stanford, CA: Stanford University Press, 2004)

Mikhalevitch, Alexandre, *Balzac et Bianchon* (Paris: Honoré Champion, 2014)

Millaud, Albert, 'Lettres fantaisistes sur Paris: M. Émile Zola', *Le Figaro*, 1 September 1876, 1–2

Miller, D. A., *The Novel and the Police* (Berkeley, CA; London: University of California Press, 1988)

Miller, Nancy K., 'Emphasis Added: Plots and Plausibilities in Women's Fiction', *PMLA*, 96.1 (1981), 36–48 <https://doi.org/10.2307/462003>

Miller, Nancy K., *The Heroine's Text: Readings in the French and English Novel, 1722–1782* (New York: Columbia University Press, 1980)

Mitterand, Henri, 'Le Quatrième Zola', *Œuvres et critiques*, 16.2 (1991), 85–98

Mossman, Carol A., *Politics and Narratives of Birth: Gynocolonization from Rousseau to Zola* (Cambridge; New York: Cambridge University Press, 1993)

Naginski, Isabelle Hoog, *George Sand: Writing for Her Life* (New Brunswick, NJ: Rutgers University Press, 1991)

O'Sullivan, Suzanne, *It's All in Your Head: True Stories of Imaginary Illness* (London: Chatto & Windus, 2015)

Otis, Laura, *Membranes: Metaphors of Invasion in Nineteenth-Century Literature, Science, and Politics* (Baltimore, MD; London: Johns Hopkins University Press, 1999)

Outka, Elizabeth, *Viral Modernism: The Influenza Pandemic and Interwar Literature* (New York: Columbia University Press, 2020)

PA Media, 'Let's Stop Clapping for the NHS, Says Woman Who Started the Ritual', *The Guardian*, 22 May 2020 <https://www.theguardian.com/world/2020/may/22/lets-stop-clapping-for-the-nhs-says-woman-who-started-the-ritual>
Patterson, Jennifer and Francia Kinchington, eds, *Body Talk in the Medical Humanities: Whose Language?* (Newcastle upon Tyne: Cambridge Scholars Publishing, 2019)
Paulson, William, 'Preceptors, Fathers, and Ideology: The Strange Narrative of Balzac's *Le Médecin de campagne*', *French Forum*, 9.1 (1984), 19–32
Petrey, Sandy, *In the Court of the Pear King: French Culture and the Rise of Realism* (Ithaca, NY: Cornell University Press, 2005)
Pierrot, Jean, *L'Imaginaire décadent (1880–1900)* (Mont-Saint-Aignan: Publications des universités de Rouen et du Havre, 2007)
Pollak, Ellen, *Incest and the English Novel, 1684–1814* (Baltimore, MD: Johns Hopkins University Press, 2003)
Poovey, Mary, 'Forgotten Writers, Neglected Histories: Charles Reade and the Nineteenth-Century Transformation of the British Literary Field', *ELH*, 71.2 (2004), 433–53
Porter, Dennis, '*Lamiel*: The Wild Child and the Ugly Men', *Novel: A Forum on Fiction*, 12.1 (1978), 21–32 <https://doi.org/10.2307/1345208>
Porter, Roy and G. S. Rousseau, *Gout: The Patrician Malady* (New Haven, CT; London: Yale University Press, 1998)
Prévost, Jean, *Essai sur les sources de 'Lamiel', les amazones de Stendhal, le procès de Lacenaire* (Lyon: Imprimeries réunies, 1942)
Przybos, Julia, 'Zola's Utopias', in *The Cambridge Companion to Émile Zola*, ed. by Brian Nelson (Cambridge: Cambridge University Press, 2007), pp. 169–87
Rabbitt, Kara M., 'L'Enfant libertine: pouvoir discursif et volonté narrative dans *Lamiel* de Stendhal', *Nineteenth Century French Studies*, 31.1 (2002), 66–83 <https://doi.org/10.1353/ncf.2002.0062>
'Rapport sur le choléra-morbus, lu à l'Académie royale de médecine, en séance générale, les 26 et 30 juillet 1831', *Journal des débats*, 18 February 1832, p. 4.
Rapport sur les épidémies cholériques de 1832 et 1849 dans les établissements dépendant de l'administration générale de l'assistance publique de la ville de Paris (Paris: Paul Dupont, 1850)
Ray, William, *Story and History: Narrative Authority and Social Identity in the Eighteenth-Century French and English Novel* (Oxford: Basil Blackwell, 1990)
Récamier, Joseph-Claude-Anthelme, *Recherches sur le traitement du choléra morbus* (Paris: Gabon, 1832)
Remein, Christy DiFrances, Ellen Childs, John Carlo Pasco, and others, 'Content and Outcomes of Narrative Medicine Programmes: A Systematic Review of the Literature through 2019', *BMJ Open*, 10.1 (2020), <https://doi.org/10.1136/bmjopen-2019-031568>
Roch, Eugène, 'Paris malade; esquisses du jour', *Journal des débats*, 29 September 1832
Rogers, Nancy, 'The Wasting Away of Romantic Heroines', *Nineteenth-Century French Studies*, 11.3/4 (1983), 246–56
Rosen, George, 'Romantic Medicine: A Problem in Historical Periodization', *Bulletin of the History of Medicine*, 25.2 (1951), 149–58
Rothfield, Lawrence, *Vital Signs: Medical Realism in Nineteenth-Century Fiction* (Princeton, NJ: Princeton University Press, 1995)
Rousseau, Jean-Jacques, *Du contrat social*, ed. by Bruno Bernardi (Paris: Flammarion, 2001)
Rousseau, Jean-Jacques, *Julie, ou la Nouvelle Héloïse*, ed. by Henri Coulet, 2 vols (Paris: Gallimard, 1993)
Rousseau, Jean-Jacques, *La Nouvelle Héloïse. Théâtre. Poésies. Essais littéraires*, ed. by Bernard Gagnebin and Marcel Raymond, in Jean-Jacques Rousseau, *Œuvres complètes*, 2 (Paris: Gallimard, 2012)
Sacks, Oliver, *The Man Who Mistook His Wife for a Hat* (London: Picador, 1986)
Sand, George, *Horace* (Paris: Hetzel et Cie; Victor Lecou, 1854)
Sand, George, *Histoire de ma vie*, ed. by Martine Reid (Paris: Gallimard, 2004)

Sand, George, *Lélia*, ed. by Pierre Reboul (Paris: Gallimard, 2003)

Sartre, Jean-Paul, *L'Être et le néant: essai d'ontologie phénoménologique*, ed. by Arlette Elkaïm-Sartre (Paris: Gallimard, 1943)

Schilling, Bernard N., *The Hero as Failure: Balzac and the Rubempré Cycle* (Chicago, IL: University of Chicago Press, 1968)

Schor, Naomi, *Breaking the Chain: Women, Theory, and French Realist Fiction* (New York: Columbia University Press, 1985)

Schor, Naomi, *George Sand and Idealism* (New York: Columbia University Press, 1993)

Schor, Naomi, *Zola's Crowds* (Baltimore, MD: Johns Hopkins University Press, 1978)

Scott, Maria, 'Performing Desire: Stendhal's Theatrical Heroines', *French Studies*, 62.3 (2008), 259–70 <https://doi.org/10.1093/fs/knn026>

Scott, Maria, 'Le Réalisme et la peur du désir? Le cas de *Lucien Leuwen*', *L'Année stendhalienne*, 9 (2010), 35–57

Scott, Maria, *Stendhal's Less-Loved Heroines: Fiction, Freedom, and the Female* (London: Legenda, 2013)

Scott, Maria, 'Stendhal's Muddy Realism', *Dix-Neuf*, 16.1 (2012), 15–27 <https://doi.org/10.1179/1478731811Z.00000000010>

Scoutetten, Henri, *Relation historique et médicale de l'épidemie de choléra qui a régné à Berlin en 1831* (Paris: J. Baillère, 1831)

Segal, Naomi, *The Adulteress's Child: Authorship and Desire in the Nineteenth-Century Novel* (Cambridge: Polity Press, 1992)

Shefer, Elaine, 'The "Bird in the Cage" in the History of Sexuality: Sir John Everett Millais and William Holman Hunt', *Journal of the History of Sexuality*, 1.3 (1991), 446–80

Shorter, Edward, 'L'Âge des premières règles en France', *Annales*, 36.3 (1981), 495–511

Showalter, Elaine, 'Hysteria, Feminism, and Gender', in Sander L. Gilman, Helen King, Roy Porter, G. S. Rousseau, and Elaine Showalter, *Hysteria Beyond Freud* (Berkeley, CA: University of California Press, 1993), pp. 286–335

Snowden, Frank M., *Epidemics and Society: From the Black Death to the Present* (New Haven, CT: Yale University Press, 2019)

Société des amis du peuple. *De la civilisation* (Paris, Carpentier de Méricourt: 1832)

Sontag, Susan, *Illness as Metaphor; and, AIDS and Its Metaphors* (London: Penguin, 1991)

Stendhal, *Correspondance générale*, ed. by Victor Del Litto, 6 vols (Paris: H. Champion, 1998), I

Stendhal, *Lucien Leuwen* (Paris: Gallimard, 2002)

Stendhal, *Œuvres romanesques complètes*, ed. by Yves Ansel, Philippe Berthier, and Xavier Bourdenet, 3 vols (Paris: Gallimard, 2005–14)

Stendhal, *Voyages en France*, ed. by Victor Del Litto (Paris: Gallimard, 1992)

Stendhal, *Voyages en Italie*, ed. by Victor Del Litto (Paris: Gallimard, 2002)

Still, Judith, *Justice and Difference in the Works of Rousseau*: Bienfaisance *and* Pudeur (Cambridge: Cambridge University Press, 1993)

Stone, Jon, 'What Should We Say to Patients with Symptoms Unexplained by Disease? The "Number Needed to Offend"', *BMJ*, 325.7378 (2002), 1449–50 <https://doi.org/10.1136/bmj.325.7378.1449>

Sylvos, Françoise, 'La Poétique de l'utopie dans *Le Médecin de campagne*', *L'Année balzacienne*, 4.1 (2003), 101–23 <https://doi.org/10.3917/balz.004.0101>

Szasz, Thomas S. and Marc Hollender, 'A Contribution to the Philosophy of Medicine: The Basic Models of the Doctor–Patient Relationship', *AMA Archives of Internal Medicine*, 97.5 (1956), 585 <https://doi.org/10.1001/archinte.1956.00250230079008>

Tacheron, Charles-François, *Statistique médicale de la mortalité du choléra-morbus dans le XIe arrondissement de Paris pendant les mois d'avril, mai, juin, juillet et août 1832* (Paris: Béchet Jeune, 1832)

Taithe, Bertrand, *Defeated Flesh: Welfare, Warfare and the Making of Modern France* (Manchester: Manchester University Press, 1999)

Tanner, Tony, *Adultery in the Novel: Contract and Transgression* (Baltimore, MD: Johns Hopkins University Press, 1981)

Ternois, René, *Zola et son temps: Lourdes, Rome, Paris* (Paris: Belles Lettres, 1961)
Testa, Carlos, 'The Sins of Utopia: Balzac's *Le Médecin de campagne*', *Nineteenth-Century French Studies*, 25 (1977), 280–92
Théodoridès, Jean, *Stendhal du côté de la science* (Aran: Éditions du Grand chêne, 1972)
Thomas, Lewis, *The Youngest Science: Notes of a Medicine-Watcher* (Oxford: Oxford University Press, 1984)
Thompson, C. W., *Lamiel, fille du feu: essai sur Stendhal et l'énergie* (Paris: L'Harmattan, 1997)
Thompson, Hannah, *Taboo: Corporeal Secrets in Nineteenth-Century France* (Oxford: Legenda, 2013)
Tilby, Michael, '*Le Médecin de campagne* et le statut du récit', *L'Année balzacienne*, 4.1 (2003), 7–24 <https://doi.org/10.3917/balz.004.0007>
Tonnellier, François, '*Le Médecin de campagne*, ou l'ambiguïté des symboles', *Les Tribunes de la santé*, 23 (2009), 57–63 <https://doi.org/10.3917/seve.023.0057>
Vigarello, Georges, *Histoire des pratiques de santé: le sain et le malsain depuis le Moyen Âge* (Paris: Points, 2016)
Viney, William, Felicity Callard, and Angela Woods, 'Critical Medical Humanities: Embracing Entanglement, Taking Risks', *Medical Humanities*, 41.1 (2015), 2–7 <https://doi.org/10.1136/medhum-2015-010692>
Waller, Margaret, *The Male Malady: Fictions of Impotence in the French Romantic Novel* (New Brunswick, NJ: Rutgers University Press, 1993).
Wettlaufer, Alexandra K., *Pen vs. Paintbrush: Girodet, Balzac, and the Myth of Pygmalion in Post-Revolutionary France* (New York: Palgrave, 2001)
White, Claire, 'Labour of Love: George Sand's *La Ville noire* and Émile Zola's *Travail*', *The Modern Language Review*, 106.3 (2011), 697–708 <https://doi.org/10.5699/modelangrevi.106.3.0697>
Whitehead, Anne, 'The Medical Humanities: A Literary Perspective', in *Medicine, Health and the Arts: Approaches to the Medical Humanities*, ed. by Victoria Bates, Alan Bleakley, and Sam Goodman (London: Routledge, 2013), pp. 107–27
Whitehead, Anne and Angela Woods, 'Introduction', in *The Edinburgh Companion to the Critical Medical Humanities*, ed. by Anne Whitehead and Angela Woods (Edinburgh: Edinburgh University Press, 2016), pp. 1–32 <https://doi.org/10.3366/edinburgh/9781474400046.003.0037>
Wilbanks, Evelyn, 'The Doctor as Romantic Hero: A Study of Idealization', *JAMA*, 220.1 (1972), 54–7 <https://doi.org/10.1001/jama.1972.03200010040006>
Wilson, Lindsay B., *Women and Medicine in the French Enlightenment: The Debate over 'maladies des femmes'* (Baltimore, MD; London: Johns Hopkins University Press, 1993)
Wilson, Steven, 'Introduction: Connecting Medicine and Religion in Modern French Literature', ed. by Steven Wilson, *Modern and Contemporary France*, L'Imaginaire médico-religieux: Modern French Literary Perspectives, 28.4 (2020), 357–64 <https://doi.org/10.1080/09639489.2020.1784860>
Wilson, Steven, *The Language of Disease: Writing Syphilis in Nineteenth-Century France* (Cambridge: Legenda, 2020)
Woods, Angela, 'Beyond the Wounded Storyteller: Rethinking Narrativity, Illness and Embodied Self-Experience', in *Health, Illness and Disease: Philosophical Essays*, ed. by Havi Carel and Rachel Cooper (London: Routledge, 2013), pp. 113–28
Woods, Angela, 'The Limits of Narrative: Provocations for the Medical Humanities', *Medical Humanities*, 37.2 (2011), 73–8 <https://doi.org/10.1136/medhum-2011-010045>
Wright, Jacinta, 'Romancing the Dead; Death and Desire in George Sand's *Lélia*', *Irish Journal of French Studies*, 1.1 (2001), 57–66 <https://doi.org/10.7173/164913301818732373>
Wright, Jacinta, '"S'habiller du vêtement du maître": George Sand et le travesti intertextuel', in *George Sand: pratiques et imaginaires de l'écriture*, ed. by Brigitte Diaz and Isabelle Hoog-Naginski, Colloques de Cerisy (Caen: Presses universitaires de Caen, 2017), 95–103
Yersin, Alexandre, 'La Peste bubonique à Hong Kong', *Annales de l'Institut Pasteur*, 8 (1894), 662–7

Zola, Émile, *Le Docteur Pascal*, ed. by Henri Mitterand (Paris: Gallimard, 2017)
Zola, Émile, *La Faute de l'abbé Mouret*, ed. by Colette Becker (Paris: Flammarion, 1999)
Zola, Émile, *Lourdes*, ed. by Jacques Noiray (Paris: Gallimard, 1995)
Zola, Émile, *Le Roman expérimental*, ed. by François-Marie Mourad (Paris: Flammarion, 2006)
Zola, Émile, *Les Rougon-Macquart*, ed. by Armand Lanoux and Henri Mitterand, 5 vols (Paris: Gallimard, 1960)

Index

For the benefit of digital users, indexed terms that span two pages (e.g., 52–53) may, on occasion, appear on only one of those pages.